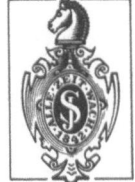

Peter I. Folb

Drug Safety
in Clinical Practice

With 24 Figures

Springer-Verlag
Berlin Heidelberg NewYork Tokyo
1984

Peter I. Folb, MD, FRCP
Professor of Pharmacology,
University of Cape Town Medical School;
Chief Physician, Groote Schuur Hospital,
Cape Town.

Library of Congress Cataloging in Publication Data
Folb, Peter I., 1938–   . Drug safety in clinical practice.
Bibliography: p. Includes index. 1. Drugs – Safety measures. 2. Drugs – Side
effects. I. Title RM301.F57 1983 615′.704283–17156
ISBN-13: 978-3-540-12811-3   e-ISBN-13: 978-1-4471-1351-5
DOI: 10.1007/ 978-1-4471-1351-5

The use of general descriptive names, trade marks, etc. in this publication, even
if the former are not to be taken as a sign that such names, as understood by
the Trade Marks and Merchandise Marks Act, may accordingly be used freely by
anyone.

Product Liability: The publisher can give no guarantee for information about
drug dosage and application thereof contained in this book. In every individual
case the respective user must check its accuracy by consulting other
pharmaceutical literature.

Filmset by Input Typesetting Limited, London, SW19 8DR

2128/3916–543210

Preface

Drugs may cause disease, or they may aggravate the morbidity of the condition for which they are prescribed, and certain patients may for one or other reason be particularly liable to drug injury. The inextricable relationships between the toxic profiles of drugs, the natural history of the diseases for which they are given, and the adverse drug effects that may develop in the course of such diseases are of considerable interest. It is the study of these rather neglected aspects of pharmacology and therapeutics which has formed the basis of this book.

An explanation is required of the approach and the style which have been followed. The monograph does not purport to be comprehensive. Only important drug groups which are commonly used in practice are considered. Emphasis has been placed on achieving maximum benefit and safety of the appropriate drugs in the management of common illnesses. When treatment fails, either *ab initio* or subsequent to an initial response, the risk-benefit relationship of drugs inevitably alters. For this reason the main factors responsible for treatment failure have been considered, with special attention to the possible contribution of or implications for drug therapy in such a situation. Finally, proposals have been put forward for improving the diagnosis and reporting of adverse drug effects.

In order to be practical and, as far as possible, constructive it has been necessary for me to "take a position" on numerous issues. In many instances I have expressed a point of view based on my understanding of authoritative literature (cited at the end of each section) and such clinical experience as I may have gained or have accrued from colleagues. There is a danger that this approach will be seen as somewhat categorical. I hope, however, that it may be understood as an attempt to depart from the descriptive and encyclopaedic approach which has tended to characterise medical writing in this particular field.

My colleagues John Straughan and Ashley Robins have in particular given me helpful advice, and I am grateful to Michael Jackson of Springer-Verlag who has guided the original idea behind the book to fruition. Renée Gelbart and June Chambers have given me much assistance in the compilation of material. Elise Fuller helped with the illustrations. The Medicines Safety Centre of the University of Cape Town Medical School, jointly sponsored by Ciba Geigy, has been a source of valuable information.

The South African Medical Research Council and the University of Cape Town have supported my researches into mechanisms and models of drug-induced damage, and this help is gratefully acknowledged.

Cape Town, 1983   Peter I. Folb

Contents

1 Drugs in Common Use

1.1 Antibiotics

The following *ground rules* for the use of antibiotics would contribute to optimising their benefit-risk relationships:

1. When adverse effects may have been experienced with previous antibiotic therapy, an alternative equally effective antibiotic of a different generic group is sought.
2. In selecting an antibiotic its clinical pharmacokinetics are considered, with special attention paid to transfer across the blood-brain barrier and distribution and elimination in renal failure and hepatic disease.
3. Combination therapy is administered only when a synergistic effect can be achieved. Unnecessary combination of antibiotics heightens the risks of toxicity, favours selection of resistant organisms, and represents additional expense, without contributing to a simpler regimen.
4. Bactericidal and bacteriostatic antibiotics are not combined (Table 1.1). This may result in a bacteriostatic effect alone, as the bactericidal activity of certain antibiotics is dependent upon rapid division of bacterial cells.
5. Antibiotics with similar toxicity profiles, which are known to cause adverse effects on the same organ, are not given together.
6. Antibiotic therapy for fever of undetermined origin is avoided as far as possible. Fever of several days' duration which is not associated with clinical signs of infection is usually due to viral infection, often of the respiratory tract, which will not respond to antibiotics. Prolonged fever, when it has an infectious cause, is most commonly due to tuberculosis or bacterial endocarditis. In either case blind use of antibiotics is likely to delay diagnosis and increase the risk of extensive damage.
7. The use of topical antibiotics (with the exception of use in the eye) is probably an important contributory factor to the development of antibiotic resistance of micro-organisms. Suitable alternatives may be effectively used for mild superficial infections. Severe skin infections are properly managed by systemic antibiotic therapy.

Table 1.1. Classification of antibiotics according to bactericidal or bacteriostatic activity (based on Reiner 1982)

Group I:	Group II:	Group III:
Bactericidal, partially also on resting micro-organisms	Bactericidal, only on proliferating micro-organisms	Bacteriostatic, in high concentrations also bactericidal
Polymyxins	Penicillin	Chloramphenicol
Streptomycin	Cephalosporins	Thiamphenicol
Neomycin	Vancomycin	Tetracyclines
Kanamycin	Rifampicin	Fusidic acid
Gentamicin		Erythromycin
Sisomicin		Lincomycin
Netilmicin		Clindamycin
Tobramycin		
Amikacin		

Notes:

1. The activity of an antibiotic combination can differ, depending on the components concerned, viz:

Indifference	—	the activity of the combination is equal to that of the more active component.
Addition	—	the activity of the combination is equal to the sum of the activities of the components.
Synergism	—	the activity of the combination is significantly greater than the sum of the components.
Antagonism	—	the activity of the combination is less than that of the more active component.

2. The combination of antibiotics *within* groups I and II usually does not display antagonism.

3. The combination of an antibiotic of group I with one of groups II or III rarely gives rise to antagonism. In general, the bactericidal agent predominates.

4. The combination of an antibiotic of group II with one of group III frequently leads to dominance of the bacteriostatic agent, i.e. the activity of the combination corresponds to the activity of the agent of group III. Antagonism is possible.

8. Prophylactic antibiotics, frequently given despite inadequate evidence that they are effective, may generate problems of toxicity and microbial resistance.

    The case for prophylaxis in rheumatic fever and bacterial endocarditis is established, and a good argument can be made for prophylaxis in meningococcal infections, diphtheria, to cover urological procedures, recurrent urinary tract infections, severe cases of chronic bronchitis, and patients with "healed" or "inactive" tuberculosis at special risk. Prophylactic antibiotics are widely used in hip replacement and vascular surgery.

9. It is important that an antibiotic is selected which has the narrowest effective range for the micro-organism or micro-organisms responsible for the infection being treated. The antibacterial range of antibiotics in common use is indicated in Fig. 1.1. For severe infections, antibiotics are ideally administered parenterally in the first instance.

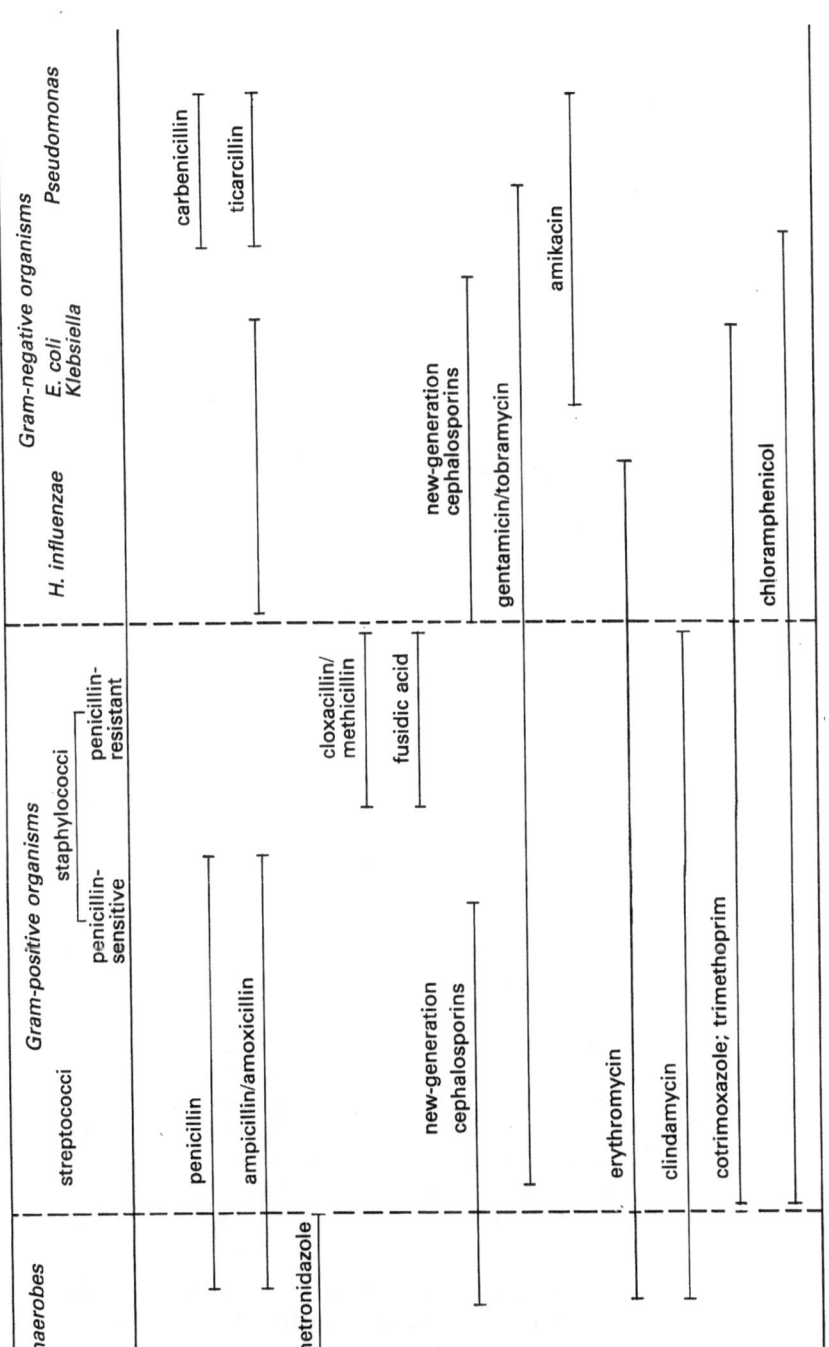

Fig. 1.1. Suggested use of common antibiotics.

TOPICAL ANTIBIOTICS

The efficacy and safety of topical application of antibiotics for infections of the skin, nares and external ear have been brought into question. For mild local infections antiseptic agents are likely to be equally effective. In severe infections the low concentrations of antibiotic achieved are unlikely to be sufficient, and systemic treatment is necessary.

There is convincing evidence that the topical use of aminoglycosides and other antibiotics such as tetracyclines and fusidic acid contributes to bacterial resistance. Suboptimal concentrations lead to selection of bacterial variants with a capacity to inactivate the drug or reduce antibiotic penetration into the bacterial cell. There may be an abrupt one-step development of resistance as a result of acquisition of extra-chromosomal DNA (plasmids). The acquired microbial resistance towards one aminoglycoside is likely to be shared by other antibiotics of the group, and not uncommonly plasmid transfer confers multiple antibiotic resistance.

As a general principle, no antibiotic which is used systemically (or is closely related to one used systemically) is applied to the surface of the body.

The eye is an exception to these general considerations. The sequelae of ocular infections may be serious, and the organisms most feared in this respect are *Pseudomonas aeruginosa*, *Streptococcus pneumoniae* and penicillin-resistant staphylococci. The penetration of agents such as sulphacetamide, chloramphenicol and gentamicin (the latter injected subconjunctivally) enable high local concentrations to be achieved.

Certain antibiotics such as the peptides (bacitracin, polymyxins and tyrocidine), polyenes (nystatin and pimaricin) and clotrimazole are not significantly absorbed from the skin or mucous membranes. They are practically free of the problems of microbial resistance; this may be attributable in part to their limited use in practice.

BETA-LACTAMASES:

β-Lactamase was originally identified as the staphylococcal enzyme capable of destroying the β-lactam ring of the penicillin nucleus, thus rendering the antibiotic inactive. With the development and widespread use of broad-spectrum, semi-synthetic penicillins and cephalosporins, penicillin- and cephalosporin-resistant Gram-negative bacteria emerged which produced a β-lactamase different to that of staphylococci. The latter is cell-bound, and confers a permeability barrier which protects the bacterial cell from antibiotic destruction. (The production of a β-lactamase in small amounts is a characteristic of many Gram-negative bacteria; it may be necessary for normal growth of the organism.)

Amongst the Gram-negative bacteria the β-lactamases can be broadly classified into:

i) Those that preferentially hydrolyse penicillins with little anti-cephalosporin activity ("penicillinases").

ii) Those that hydrolyse cephalosporins with little anti-penicillin activity ("cephalosporinases").

iii) "Broad-spectrum" β-lactamases that hydrolyse both penicillins and cephalosporins to a considerable extent.

Most penicillinases destroy benzylpenicillin, penicillin V, ampicillin, amoxicillin and carbenicillin. No β-lactam antibiotic is completely resistant to the β-lactamases. The degree of penicillinase and cephalosporinase production of various micro-organisms is indicated in Table 1.2.

Table 1.2. β-Lactamase production by various micro-organisms

	Penicillinase	Cephalosporinase[a]
Staph. aureus	++++	+++ →+
Ps. aeruginosa	++++	++ →+
Proteus sp.	+++	+ →+
Haemophilus influenzae	++++	+++ →+
Klebsiella sp.	++++	++ →+
Bacteroides fragilis	++++	++++→+

[a]The cephalosporinases are less effective against the new-generation cephalosporins.

SIDE-EFFECTS

A distinction can be made between (a) dose-related adverse effects that are predictable from the pharmacological action and toxicity profile of an antibiotic or from biological effects due to growth inhibition of the normal bacterial flora, such as is frequently encountered with broad-spectrum antibiotics, and (b) allergic reactions, which are dose-independent and in the main not predictable.

A profile of side-effects of different antibiotics and chemotherapeutic agents is given in Table 1.3.

Table 1.3. Side-effects of antibiotics and chemotherapeutic agents

Antibiotic or chemotherapeutic agent	Side-effects					Contra-indicated or to be used with considerable caution in advanced renal insufficiency
	Allergic	Haemato-toxic	Nephrotoxic	Hepatotoxic	Neurotoxic	
Penicillin	++[1]				+	
Flucloxacillin; dicloxacillin	++				±	
Amoxicillin; ampicillin	++				±	
New cephalosporins	+[1]	±				
Chloramphenicol	±	+[2]			±	
Aminoglycosides[3]	+		+[4]		++[5]	X
Tetracyclines	±	±		±		X[6]
Erythromycin; clindamycin[7]	±			±		
Fusidic acid	±					
Vancomycin	++		+		+	X
Sulphonamides; cotrimoxazole	++	±	±	±		

Key: ± = rare; + = uncommon; ++ = relatively frequent
Numbers refer to the following notes

Notes:

1. For discussion of allergic reactions to the penicillins and cephalosporins refer to p. 00.
2. Chloramphenicol depresses the bone marrow by one of two mechanisms:
   i) A dose-related reversible effect mainly on the formation of red cells, but at times also platelets and granulocytes; and
   ii) Severe aplasia with pancytopenia, which is uncommon, unpredictable, not dose-related, and idiosyncratic.

   The former appears to be due to inhibition of mitochondrial protein synthesis. The latter probably results from a genetically determined biochemical predisposition (a defect in nucleic acid synthesis has been suggested).

3. The comparative toxicity of the aminoglycosides is set out below:

Antibiotic	Effects on:			
	Vestibulum	Cochlea	Kidney	Neuromuscular blocking
Streptomycin	+++	+	+	++
Dihydrostreptomycin	+	+++	+	+
Neomycin	+	++++	+++	+++
Framycetin	+	++++	+++	+++
Kanamycin	+	+++	++	+++
Gentamicin	++	+	++	++
Tobramycin	++	+	++	++

4. The risk of aminoglycoside nephrotoxicity is greater in the following circumstances: concomitant treatment with other potentially nephrotoxic antibiotics (e.g. vancomycin); treatment in excess of 10–14 days; serious coexistent disease such as coagulopathy, bleeding, shock, dehydration and urate nephropathy (in cancer patients on cytotoxic treatment).

5. The aminoglycosides destroy the sensory hair cells in the inner ear (organ of Corti of the cochlea). The risk of aminoglycoside ototoxicity is greater with concomitant use of high-ceiling diuretics, usage in excess of 10 days, renal disease with decompensation, high dosage, recent aminoglycoside therapy, pre-existing ear disease and in patients older than 40 years.

   Delayed ototoxicity may occur even after treatment has been discontinued. This is thought to be due to the persistent toxic effect of accumulated drug in the inner ear and semicircular canals. Unilateral aminoglycoside ototoxicity has been described. Topically administered aminoglycosides in the ear may account for some deafness complicating otitis media.

   Even the "non-absorbable" aminoglycosides such as neomycin can be absorbed from the gastrointestinal tract or following intrabronchial or intraperitoneal administration in sufficient amounts to cause deafness. This is likely when there is coexistent renal insufficiency and the antibiotic cannot be normally eliminated.

6. Doxycycline can be administered in renal insufficiency, although appropriate dosage adjustments are necessary in advanced failure (see Table 1.4), and because of poor filtration into the urine it is unlikely to be effective in urinary tract infections in such patients. (Between 60% and 70% of the other tetracyclines is excreted in the urine; 35%–40% of a dose of doxycycline is excreted in the urine.)

7. A serious potential side-effect of clindamycin therapy is pseudomembranous colitis.

RENAL ELIMINATION

Many antimicrobial agents are eliminated primarily by the kidneys. The aminoglycosides, the polymyxins and vancomycin are exclusively eliminated by renal mechanisms and their toxicity correlates directly with concentrations in plasma and tissues. Since the adverse effects of these antibiotics involve the kidneys a vicious cycle may develop if they accumulate in the body.

Tetracyclines accumulate in patients with impaired renal function, with the exception of doxycycline. Uraemia may be aggravated by the catabolic effect of elevated amounts of tetracycline.

A guideline for dosage adjustments for patients in renal failure is given in Table 1.4.

HEPATIC DISEASE AND FAILURE

The dosage of antibiotics excreted by the liver (erythromycin, chloramphenicol, lincomycin, clindamycin and doxycycline) must be reduced in patients with hepatic failure.

If there is infection in the biliary tract, hepatic disease or biliary obstruction may reduce access of an antibiotic to the site of the infection. This has been shown to occur with several drugs normally excreted in the bile.

Table 1.4. Dosage guidelines for antibiotic therapy in renal failure [reproduced with kind permission from Bennett W. M. et al. (1980) Drug therapy in renal failure. Ann Intern Med 93:62]

Antibiotic	Major excretion route[a]	Normal time of elimination (h)	ESRD[b]	Normal dose interval (h)	Adjustment for renal failure: creatinine clearance[c]		
					>50	10–50	<10
Penicillin G	Renal	0.5	6–20	8	Nil	75% of dose	
Ampicillin/ amoxicillin	Renal (hepatic)	1.5	7–20	6	Nil	6–12 h intervals	12–16 h intervals
Cephamandole	Renal	1.0	11	4–6	Nil	25% –50% normal dose	25% normal dose
Cloxacillin	Hepatic (renal)	0.4–0.6	0.8	6		Nil	
Carbenicillin	Renal (hepatic)	1.5	10–20	2–4	Dose at 8–12 h intervals	12–24 h intervals	24–48 h intervals
Gentamicin/ tobramycin	Renal	2.0	24–48	8	Dose at 12 h intervals	Dose at 12–48 h intervals	Dose at 48–72 h intervals
Chloramphenicol	Hepatic (renal)	2.5	3–7	6		Nil	
Doxycycline	Renal (hepatic)	14–25	15–37	12	Nil	Dose at 12–18 h intervals	Dose at 18–24 h intervals
Sulphamethoxazole/ trimethoprim	Renal	Sulph. 9–11	24			Dose at 18 h intervals	Dose at 24 h intervals
		Trim. 8–15	20–50	12	Nil		
Metronidazole	Hepatic	6–14	8–15	8	Nil	Nil	Dose at 12 h intervals

[a]Alternative, significant routes of elimination are indicated in parentheses
[b]ESRD = end stage renal disease
[c]Expressed as ml/min

FURTHER READING

Editorial (1978) Antibiotic resistance and topical treatment. Br Med J II: 649
Keller H. Bircher J (1980) Miscellaneous antibiotics. In: Dukes MNG (ed) Meyler's side effects of drugs, 9th edn. Excerpta Medica, Amsterdam, p. 452
Kucers A, Bennet N McK (1979) The use of antibiotics, 3rd edn. Heinemann, London
Reiner R. (1982) Antibiotics. An introduction. Thieme, Stuttgart

1.2 Antihistamines

The antihistamines are widely used in the treatment and prophylaxis of motion sickness (where they are valuable), to produce sedation (where they are effective), for allergic conditions (effective), and for symptomatic relief of colds and upper respiratory tract infections characterised by rhinorrhoea and excessive secretions (where their efficacy has not been established).

They have a wide therapeutic margin, which no doubt accounts for their excessive and often inappropriate use. They are active constituents of many over-the-counter proprietary medicines.

Antihistamines blocking H_1-receptors fall into one of the following chemical groups: ethanolamines, alkylamines, ethylenediamines, piperazines and phenothiazines.

USE IN THE COMMON COLD AND UPPER RESPIRATORY TRACT INFECTIONS

In the common cold and other upper respiratory tract infections scientific evidence in support of efficacy is lacking. On the contrary, antihistamines may have an atropine-like drying effect, leading to inspissation of sputum, and possibly to the development of otitis media and middle ear effusion as a result of the effects on mucociliary action affecting paranasal sinuses and eustachian tubes.

Antihistamines are often present in combined products such as expectorants and cough suppressants and with sympathomimetic agents designed for the symptomatic treatment of coughs, colds and respiratory tract infections.

SPECIAL PROBLEMS

i) The elderly are at particular risk from the adverse effects of antihistamines, which regularly cause sedation, drowsiness or dizziness, and sometimes excitation, euphoria, confusion or nervousness. These central nervous system effects could be due to a central anticholinergic action.

ii) Glaucoma, prostatism or urinary retention may be aggravated by the anticholinergic effects of these agents.

iii) Tachycardia and hypertension have occasionally been reported with various antihistamines, which should be used with caution in patients with cardiac disease or hypertension.

iv) Motor vehicle drivers and those operating

machinery or required to climb heights may be at danger due to the sedative effects, impairment of psychomotor activity and the blurring of vision which may be caused by antihistamines. These effects are greatest at the initiation of treatment. (See section on drugs and driving, p. 149).

v) Reference is made in the section on drug usage in pregnancy (p. 135) to the risk of antihistamines to the fetus.

vi) Antihistamines should be avoided in patients with advanced liver disease as they may precipitate coma. The antihistamines are mainly metabolised in the liver.

vii) In renal failure the dosage of certain antihistamines requires adjustment to obviate accumulation and toxicity (Table 1.5).

Table 1.5. Dosage adjustments of antihistamines in renal failure [based on Heel RC, Avery GS (1980) Guide to drug dosage in renal failure. In: Avery GS (ed) Drug treatment. Adis, Balgowlah, Australia, p 1290]

Drug	Normal elimination half-life (h)	Percentage excreted unchanged in urine	Normal extra-renal mode of excretion	Normal dose interval (h)	Dose adjustment for renal failure[a]			Toxic effects in renal failure
					>50	10–50	<10	
Chlorpheniramine	±30	10–30	Not known	4–6	Unch.	Unch.	Unch.	Sedation
Diphenhydramine	4–10	4	Hepatic	6	6	6–9	9–12	Sedation; acute urinary retention in the elderly
Promethazine	Not known	Not known	Not known	12	12	12–18	18–24	As above, also anticholinergic activity

Key: Unch. = unchanged
[a]According to creatinine clearance

INTERACTION WITH OTHER DRUGS

Given with other central nervous system depressants, particularly alcohol, there may be marked potentiation of the sedative effect of the antihistamines. Important in this regard are the tricyclic antidepressants, barbiturates, benzodiazepines, β-blockers and non-barbiturate sedatives.

Such sedation may represent a danger for the patient in terms of ability to drive a motor car and other aspects of psychomotor activity.

ADVERSE EFFECTS ON
THE NERVOUS SYSTEM

Depression of the central nervous system is the commonest adverse effect of the H_1-antagonists. Tolerance to this may develop after several days' use. The sedative effect of antihistamines seems to be an unpleasant experience for most individuals. Other adverse central nervous effects include dizziness, lassitude, incoordination, fatigue, blurred vision, diplopia, euphoria, nervousness, insomnia and tremor.

There is individual variation in these responses depending upon the drug (ethanolamines are particularly likely to produce central nervous system effects), and pharmacokinetic differences. Limiting dosing to night-time may reduce these unwanted effects.

Central nervous system stimulation may complicate the use of antihistamines, in the form of insomnia, irritability and tremor. Nightmares and hallucinations have been reported. All the H_1-blockers may produce anticholinergic side-effects including erectile problems and diminution of sexual desire. Adverse effects of pharmacological doses attributable to anticholinergic activity are dryness of the mouth, pharynx and tracheobronchial tree, nasal stuffiness, blurring of vision with impaired colour discrimination and night vision, urinary retention, constipation, nausea, vomiting and epigastric discomfort.

The anticholinergic toxicity of the antihistamines may differ according to the class of agent (Table 1.6).

TOPICAL USE

Anaesthetic activity of topically applied antihistamines diminishes pruritus, but their efficacy in allergy has not been demonstrated. Locally applied antihistamines are likely to produce skin sensitisation and contact dermatitis. The ethylenediamines and phenothiazines are also capable of causing photoallergic cutaneous reactions.

Topical administration in sufficient doses can result in systemic absorption and toxicity.

The Committee on Drugs of The American Academy of Pediatrics has made the following recommendations:

　i) To discontinue the use of topical antihistamine

Table 1.6. Anticholinergic activity and toxicity of the antihistamines (H₁-antagonists)

Class of H₁-blocking drugs	Prototype	Antimuscarinic activity	Profile of antimuscarinic side-effects
Ethanolamines	Diphenhydramine	Significant	The incidence of gastro-intestinal side-effects is low in this group
Ethylenediamines	Pyrilamine	?	Gastrointestinal side-effects are common in this group
Alkylamines	Chlorpheniramine	Not significant	–
Piperazines	Chlorcyclizine	Anticholinergic effects are less than with other H₁-blocking drugs	Anticholinergic side-effects may nevertheless be disturbing
Phenothiazines	Promethazine	Considerable	Anticholinergic effects may be disabling

preparations because their toxicity is believed to exceed their limited advantages.

ii) Patients should be discouraged from purchasing over-the-counter topical antihistamine preparations.

iii) The frequency of contact dermatitis from antihistaminic agents should be kept in mind in the evaluation of dermatitis of unknown aetiology.

ACUTE POISONING

The antihistamines have a relatively high margin of safety, but acute poisoning is nevertheless common.

Central nervous system depression is the rule; in children stimulation is common. Anticholinergic features are characteristic. Deepening coma with cardiorespiratory collapse and death usually occurs within 2–18 h in the worst cases (see Fig. 1.2).

FURTHER READING

American Academy of Pediatrics, Committee on Drugs (1973) Antihistamines in topical preparations. Pediatrics 51: 299
British National Formulary (1981) No. 1. British Medical Association and The Pharmaceutical Society of Great Britain, London, p 261
Burks TF (1979) Neuropsychiatric side effects of drugs in the elderly. In: Levenson AF (ed) Ageing, vol 9. Raven, New York, p 69

Douglas WW (1980) H₁-blocking agents. In: Goodman LS, Gilman AG, Gilman A (eds) The pharmacological basis of therapeutics, 6th edn. Macmillan, New York, p 626

Fastner Z (1980) Antihistamines. In: Dukes MNG (ed) Meyler's side effects of drugs, 9th edn. Excerpta Medica, Amsterdam, p 265

Federal Register, Food and Drug Administration (1971) OTC topical antihistamines; drug efficacy study. 36: 18021

Peerless SA, Noiman AH (1980) Etiology of otitis media with effusion; antihistamine-decongestants. Laryngoscope 90: 1852

1.3 Histamine₂-Receptor Blocking Agents

Histamine₂ (H₂)-receptors are identifiable in the gastric mucosa, central nervous system, and heart and cardiovascular system, although their biological significance in the latter is not clear. Antagonists to the H₂-receptors, pre-eminently cimetidine, have been widely and successfully used to inhibit gastric acid secretion induced by cholinergic stimuli, and they have proved to be effective in the treatment of peptic ulceration. They are marginally superior to antacids in this regard. H₂-receptor antagonists have also been used to protect seriously ill patients from acute upper gastrointestinal bleeding; antacids are better for this purpose, and such patients appear to be at greatest risk of toxicity from these agents.

CIMETIDINE

Cimetidine readily crosses the blood-brain barrier, and encephalopathy due to cimetidine is a prominent adverse effect. The manifestations range from mental confusion, agitation, delirium (which may simulate delirium tremens), hallucinations, and myoclonus to coma and epilepsy. These resemble a toxic confusional state or organic brain syndrome. They may be due to H₂-receptor blockade in the central nervous system, or, alternatively, the result of a central anticholinergic action. (An anti-H₂ action may be a common mechanism whereby amitriptyline, promethazine and cimetidine produce adverse neuropsychiatric symptoms; all are antagonistic for H₂-receptors in vitro.)

The neurotoxicity of cimetidine is dose-related and correlates with serum levels of the drug. It is most commonly seen in patients of advanced age, and with impaired renal function. Hepatic cirrhosis, liver failure, concomitant serious medical illness and combined use of cimetidine with other CNS-depressant drugs are contributory factors. In combined hepatic and renal failure the half-life of elimination of cimetidine may be ten times the normal value of 2 h.

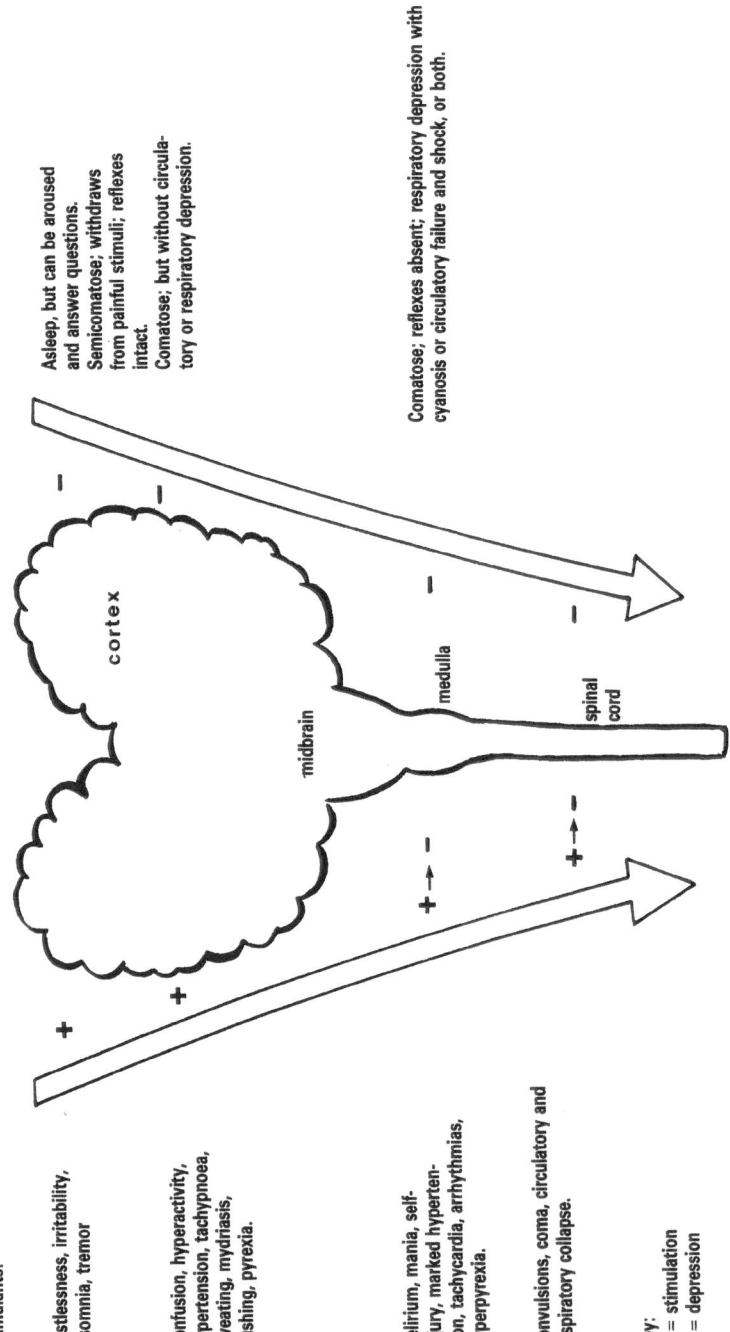

Stimulants:

Restlessness, irritability, insomnia, tremor

Confusion, hyperactivity, hypertension, tachypnoea, sweating, mydriasis, flushing, pyrexia.

Delirium, mania, self-injury, marked hypertension, tachycardia, arrhythmias, hyperpyrexia.

Convulsions, coma, circulatory and respiratory collapse.

Key:
+ = stimulation
− = depression

Depressants

Asleep, but can be aroused and answer questions.
Semicomatose; withdraws from painful stimuli; reflexes intact.
Comatose; but without circulatory or respiratory depression.

Comatose; reflexes absent; respiratory depression with cyanosis or circulatory failure and shock, or both.

Fig. 1.2. Signs and symptoms of intoxication of CNS depressants and stimulants.
[Based on Gilman AG, Goodman LS, Gilman A (eds) (1980) The pharmacological basis of therapeutics, 6th edn. Macmillan, New York; Plum F, Posner JB (1980) Diagnosis of stupor and coma, 3rd edn. Davis, Philadephia]

A depressive syndrome associated with cimetidine has been described; this may represent another form of neurotoxicity of the drug.

The main metabolite of cimetidine can produce increased prolactin levels leading to gynaecomastia in males and galactorrhoea in females. The drug probably induces prolactin release from the pituitary, but inhibition of peripheral prolactin uptake is also possible.

Cimetidine is a potent inhibitor of hepatic microsomal enzyme activity, and it may *inter alia* diminish metabolism of the benzodiazepines, diazepam and chlordiazepoxide, prolonging their elimination half-life. (This inhibition can occur within hours.) When cimetidine is administered concurrently with other drugs which have a depressant action on the central nervous system, particularly when these are dependent on hepatic microsomal enzymes for elimination, a synergistic action may result.

Several guidelines can be defined for improving the safe use of cimetidine:

i) The dosage should be adjusted in elderly patients or in patients suffering from renal and/or hepatic failure, in order to reduce the risk of mental confusion (in renal failure the maximum daily dose should not exceed 400 mg).

ii) For patients who develop cimetidine-associated changes in mental status and in whom treatment cannot be discontinued, the dose and frequency of administration should be individualised.

iii) When a benzodiazepine has to be administered at the same time, those benzodiazepines which have a short half-life of elimination and which are not metabolised in the liver (such as oxazepam or lorazepam) are preferred.

RANITIDINE

Ranitidine is an H₂-receptor antagonist which was developed subsequent to cimetidine. It is more water-soluble than its predecessor and is thought to be less likely to cross the blood-brain barrier. However, the clinical implications of this difference in drug distribution will have to be rigorously

examined in practice, particularly in patients at
special risk, before judgement can be passed as to
the comparative safety of the two agents.

FURTHER READING

Priebe HJ et al. (1980) Cimetidine in preventing acute gastrointestinal bleeding. N Engl J Med
    302:426
Schentag JJ et al. (1981) Cimetidine disposition. Clin Pharmacol Ther 29:737
Smitz S et al. (1982) Cimetidine neurotoxicity and anticholinergic activity. Am J Psychiatry
    139:704

1.4 Antacids

Antacids in effective dosage are neutralisers of gastric acidity, but their
capacity for relief of pain in peptic ulceration is not superior to placebo. Ulcer
healing can be shown to be promoted by antacids: the healing rate of duodenal
ulcers and gastric ulcers at 6 weeks has been significantly better than that of
placebo in various studies.

Large-dose, prolonged antacid therapy in peptic ulceration may be associated
with several complications:

ALUMINIUM TOXICITY   Excessive intake of aluminium-containing antacids
(with the exception of aluminium phosphate) may
cause phosphate trapping in the intestine due to
the formation of insoluble aluminium phosphate.
Faecal loss of phosphate, and the hypophosphataemia which may result, cause leaching of calcium
from bones, hypophosphaturia and consequent
over-production of 1α-dihydroxy-vitamin D_2. The
latter is a potent stimulus to osteoclastic activity,
further promoting calcium loss from bone (Fig.
1.3).

The effects of chronic hypophosphataemia (phosphorus depletion syndrome) are debility, anorexia,
malaise, muscle weakness, bone pain and hyper-
calciuria. Osteomalacia and pseudofractures may
develop as a result of demineralisation of bone.
Symptoms may be aggravated when dietary intake
of phosphorus is low, as is often the case in patients on a low protein diet.

The true incidence of aluminium-induced bone
disease is not known, but it is likely that antacid-
induced hypophosphataemia will increase in the

future. Diets with high phosphorus content (milk, peanuts, red meat, egg, fish and cheddar cheese) are used less commonly in the routine management of peptic ulcer disease, and antacids are being recommended in larger doses than in the past. Routine serum chemistry investigations in hospital practice commonly include calcium and phosphorus, making it probable that the syndrome will be recognised more often than in the past.

CHRONIC ALUMINIUM
TOXICITY

Although aluminium is widely believed to be non-toxic, poorly absorbed, and excreted in the faeces as a result of formation of insoluble complexes with phosphate in the intestine, evidence is accumulating that it is in fact absorbed in significant amounts from the gut, and that it localises in certain tissues.

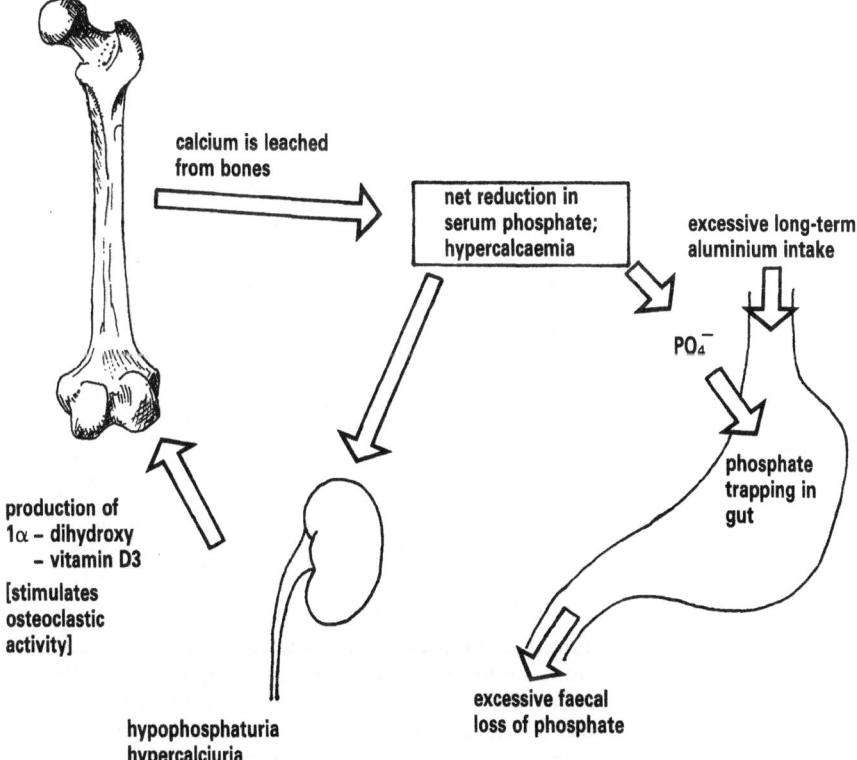

Fig. 1.3. Consequences of long-term ingestion of aluminium-containing antacids

Normal plasma aluminium levels may be elevated two-fold with regular aluminium hydroxide intake, and considerably higher levels have been reported in patients with renal failure treated for prolonged periods. Levels of aluminium 10–20 times normal have been found post mortem in the cerebral cortex of such patients, and it has been suggested that aluminium may have a pathogenic role in dialysis dementia. It may be that aluminium accumulates in the brain as a result of permeability of the blood-brain barrier in renal failure. (In at least two other investigations the aluminium content of the cerebral cortex of patients with dialysis dementia was not significantly different from that of patients dying in renal failure without dementia.)

BISMUTH
ENCEPHALOPATHY AND
NEUROPATHY

Insoluble bismuth salts are used as protective agents for the gastric and duodenal lining in the treatment of peptic ulceration. Bismuth subgallate has been used to control the odour and consistency of the stool in colostomy or ileostomy patients. Trivalent insoluble bismuth salts are used to control diarrhoea. Bismuth preparations have very weak antacid properties.

Although bismuth is poorly absorbed from the gastrointestinal tract, bismuth subnitrate and subgallate have caused clinical toxicity associated with high plasma bismuth levels. Once absorbed it diffuses into the tissues, and achieves comparatively high concentrations in the kidney, which is the major organ of excretion.

Bismuth intoxication has been reported from Australia, where the subgallate form was widely used in the management of post-colostomy and ileostomy patients, and from France, where bismuth subnitrate was extensively used as an antacid. Poisoning has also been described following long-term topical application of a bismuth and mercury bleach cream.

The neurological symptoms described are confusion, tremulousness, clumsiness, myoclonic jerks, paraesthesiae, impairment of concentration and other intellectual functions, dementia, hallucinations, convulsions, psychosis and peripheral neuropathy.

Early in the treatment it may be difficult to recognise bismuth encephalopathy, as the symptoms can be obscure. A characteristic complaint is insomnia. The encephalopathic effects appear to correlate with serum levels of bismuth, although impairment of intellect may be permanent.

It is not certain whether the chronic administration of bismuth as an antacid causes these complications. However, because of lack of clarity concerning long-term safety and their dubious efficacy as antacids, numerous authorities regard bismuth-containing preparations as obsolete.

Other problems associated with antacids include nausea and vomiting caused by aluminium, which are due to its local astringent action in the upper gastrointestinal tract, and constipation, which is regularly associated with its use; magnesium on the other hand causes diarrhoea, and this may be used to offset the effects of the former. Magnesium is absorbed from the bowel, with possible toxic consequences in patients with renal failure. Calcium-containing antacids may cause renal damage due to alkalosis and hypercalcaemia. Antacids with a high sodium content may exceed normal daily requirements of sodium by a factor of 20. Patients with sodium-retaining states may be put at serious risk as a result.

The absorption of other drugs such as antibiotics, digoxin, anticonvulsants, warfarin and anti-inflammatory drugs may be altered when they are taken together with antacids, although supporting evidence in this connection has not always been very clear.

FURTHER READING

Arieff AI et al. (1979) Aluminium toxicity. Ann Intern Med 90:741
Editorial (1981) Antacids for duodenal ulcer. Br Med J 282:1495
Fastner Z (1980) Metals. In: Dukes MNG (ed) Meyler's side effects of drugs, 9th edn. Excerpta Medica, Amsterdam, p 368
Hurwitz A (1977) Antacid therapy and drug kinetics. Clin Pharmacokinetics 2:269
Spencer H, Lender M (1979) Aluminium toxicity. Gastroenterology 76:603

1.5 Laxatives

Laxatives act to promote evacuation of the bowel. The differences between laxatives, cathartics and purgatives are of degree. Large doses of a laxative may produce a cathartic effect.

Millions of people who use laxatives do not really need them. There are few valid indications for their use for longer than 1 week. The use of laxatives for undiagnosed abdominal pain, vomiting, possible acute appendicitis and other digestive symptoms can lead to serious complications.

SAFETY PROFILES

Bulk-forming laxatives (e.g. dietary bran, cellulose derivatives, malt soup extract) are among the safest. They are not absorbed from the digestive tract and they soften and increase the frequency of stools by holding water in the bowel. These preparations are dry, and a liberal intake of fluids is necessary. Bulk laxatives may be contraindicated in patients with ulcerative colitis, regional ileitis or partial intestinal obstruction.

The *anthraquinones* (aloe, cascara sagrada, senna, etc.) are safe and effective when taken in appropriate amounts for occasional use. With excessive use, or in overdose, effects such as diarrhoea with metabolic acidosis, muscle weakness due to hypokalaemia, and metabolic alkalosis may occur.

Bisacodyl appears to act by inhibiting the sodium pump, thus stimulating the secretion into the intestine of potassium, and in this way effecting increased fluid movement into the lumen. In excess, bisacodyl may cause the "cathartic syndrome".

CATHARTIC SYNDROME

The cathartic syndrome may develop as a result of chronic laxative ingestion, overt or surreptitious. Several watery motions are likely to be passed each day, resulting in diarrhoea, abdominal discomfort (sometimes pain), muscle weakness, lassitude, and electrolyte disturbances, particularly hypokalaemia. Fluid loss may amount to 2 l a day—a potent cause of dehydration. Sodium concentrations in diarrhoeal stools of this magnitude may approach those of the plasma (100–140 mEq/1 of stool), and this will rapidly lead to sodium depletion.

Sigmoidoscopy and barium meal examination may reveal evidence of the "cathartic colon"—pathological superficial mucosal epithelial changes in the colon and rectum with inflammatory changes resembling ulcerative proctitis or colitis, and radiological evidence of dilated, abnormally distensile and hypomotile colon with poor or absent haustral markings. "Pseudostrictures" may be noted (i.e. areas of colonic spasm that persist for several hours).

CHRONIC
HYPOKALAEMIA

With excessive purgation, losses of potassium may be of the order of 5–15 mEq/1 of stool. This potassium loss is not directly accountable by stool loss; a contributory factor in certain instances may be through secondary hyperaldosteronism. Persistent hypokalaemia may have severe long-term effects. The renal tubules are particularly vulnerable, and chronic renal failure may develop.

MINERAL OIL DEPOSITS

Repeated oral administration of mineral oil may result in accumulation of lipid in the liver, spleen and lymph nodes. Such deposits need not necessarily be harmful, but if oil gains access to the lungs a lipoid pneumonitis is likely to result. There is a greater danger of this if it is taken at bedtime, and the risk is highest in elderly, debilitated or dysphagic individuals.

Leakage of the oil past the anal sphincter may cause pruritus ani. Continuous presence of oil in the rectum disturbs defaecatory reflexes, and may interfere with healing of postoperative wounds in the anorectal region.

Other adverse effects caused by laxatives include a steatorrhoeic syndrome as a result of chronic abuse, thought to be due to impairment of small intestinal function; osteomalacia, due to malabsorption of calcium, presumably also caused by a small intestinal defect; and excessive absorption of magnesium from magnesium-containing laxatives which in sufficient quantities, and particularly in patients with impaired renal function, can cause cerebral irritation, coma, respiratory depression, muscle paralysis and cardiac arrhythmias.

PHENOLPHTHALEIN

A large number of laxative preparations contain phenolphthalein, of which some are also used for reduction of body mass or in combination with other agents such as analgesics. There is no evidence that phenolphthalein is effective for these other purposes.

Phenolphthalein has an acidic structure (Fig. 1.4) and when taken in massive doses it may give rise to severe metabolic acidosis, with acute renal failure. More commonly, phenolphthalein causes a spectrum of toxic allergic skin reactions ranging from a fixed drug reaction to erythema multiforme and toxic epidermal necrolysis. The latter may be life threatening. The epidermal reactions to phenolphthalein may be idiosyncratic or of the toxic type, predictable and dose-related.

There is no evidence that yellow phenolphthalein, which is less pure and more potent than the white form, is more likely than the latter to cause toxic and allergic reactions. The overall incidence of adverse reactions to phenolphthalein is low, but considering its widespread use they are not unimportant.

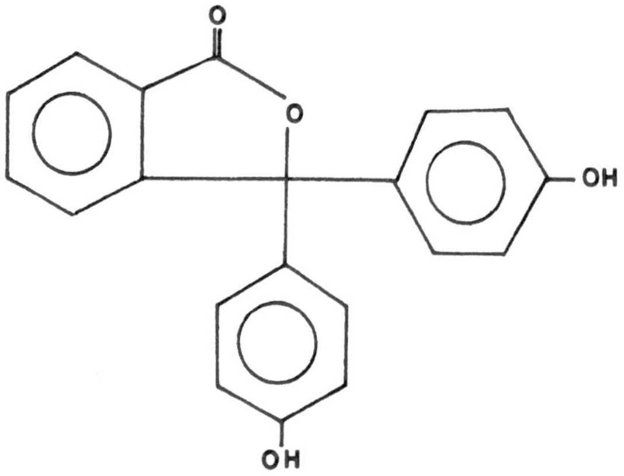

Fig. 1.4. The structure of phenolphthalein.

FURTHER READING

Cooke WR (1977) Laxative abuse. Clin Gastroenterol 6:659
Cummings JH (1974) Laxative-induced diarrhoea. Gut 15:758
Federal Register, Food and Drug Administration (1975) Constipation and the use of over the counter laxatives. 40(56):12904
Meisel JL et al. (1977) Rectal pathology. Gastroenterology 72:1274

1.6 Antidiarrhoeal Agents

Many of the antidiarrhoeal agents, with the exception of the opiates and diphenoxylate, have yet to be submitted to properly controlled clinical trials to establish their efficacy. They are, nonetheless, widely used.

KAOLIN   Kaolin is a natural hydrated aluminium silicate.

The supposed ability of this chemical to adsorb bacteria and toxins has not been proven, and neither has its efficacy as an antidiarrhoeal agent. In the doses in which it is normally used kaolin can be regarded as safe. It is possible (but has not been shown) that kaolin may adsorb to other drugs in the gut (e.g. cardiac glycosides, antibiotics and vitamins), reducing their bioavailability.

PECTIN

Pectin, a purified carbohydrate product obtained from the rind of citrus fruits or from apple pomace, is safe in doses taken orally. However, little evidence exists of its efficacy. Kaopectin is a popular product which contains 25% kaolin and 1% pectin.

BISMUTH

Bismuth subsalicylate is safe in amounts taken orally for diarrhoea, but there are questions regarding the safety of bismuth subnitrate. Large doses of the latter have caused methaemoglobinaemia in infants, as a result of absorption of nitrate, and for this reason it is contraindicated in children under 2 years. There is little evidence to support the effectiveness of bismuth salts in diarrhoea.

ANTICHOLINERGICS

By reducing gastrointestinal motility and tone anticholinergic agents such as atropine, tincture of belladonna and propantheline bromide may be of benefit in intestinal spasm and pain. There is no evidence that the small quantities of anticholinergic agents normally present in antidiarrhoeal products contribute to their effectiveness. Furthermore, these agents have the potential for toxicity, especially in young children (see p. 175).

OPIATES

Morphine and codeine are effective antidiarrhoeals. There is the hazard of addiction with prolonged use. Opiates cause high intraluminal pressure, which is a possible pathogenic factor in diverticular disease, and the latter is a contraindication to their use.

DIPHENOXYLATE AND ATROPINE

The combination of diphenoxylate and atropine is generally known by the proprietary name, Lomotil. Diphenoxylate has gastrointestinal properties similar to the opiates but with less addiction potential. To minimise abuse of diphenoxylate a subtherapeutic dose of atropine has been added. This combination has to be avoided in patients with chronic liver disease since hepatic coma may be precipitated. Children under the age of 2 years may be extremely sensitive to the depressant effects of diphenoxylate on the central nervous system. The drug is contraindicated in this age group. Signs of intoxication may resemble atropinism.

IODOCHLORHYDROXY-QUIN

Iodochlorhydroxyquin (clioquinol) was found in the early 1970s in Japan to be associated with subacute myelo-optic neuropathy (SMON). A syndrome like SMON has also been described in patients in Europe and the United States who have taken iodochlorhydroxyquin. This agent has been withdrawn from the American market, but it remains available in numerous other countries. It is not known whether the drug is associated with SMON when it is taken in standard doses for acute diarrhoeal disease, and neither has it been adequately documented as effective in appropriate trials.

ANTIDIARRHOEAL / ANTIBIOTIC COMBINATIONS

The rationale for antidiarrhoeal agents containing an antibiotic is not scientifically justifiable. Most diarrhoeal illnesses are self-limiting and do not require antibiotics. Many are viral and do not require antimicrobial therapy. Furthermore, antibiotics encourage the emergence of resistant bacterial strains, and bowel superinfection. In severe bacterial infection systemic administration of an antibiotic is essential.

These comments refer equally to the sulphonamides.

FURTHER READING

Federal Register, Food and Drug Administration (1975) Antidiarrhoeal agents. 40(56):12924
Medical Letter on Drugs and Therapeutics (1975) Iodochlorhydroxyquin. 17:105
Pietrusco RG (1979) Drug therapy reviews: pharmacotherapy of diarrhoea. Am J Hosp Pharm 36:757

1.7 Aspirin and the Acidic Non-steroidal Anti-inflammatory Agents

These drugs, which inhibit prostaglandin synthesis and have in common analgesic, antipyretic and anti-inflammatory properties, share a toxicity profile. Considerable variation exists in patients' responses to the anti-inflammatory and analgesic actions of these agents, and to their toxic effects. The reasons are not understood.

The following side-effects may be seen with aspirin or with any of the non-steroidal acidic anti-inflammatory agents (NSAIAs) shown in Fig. 1.5.

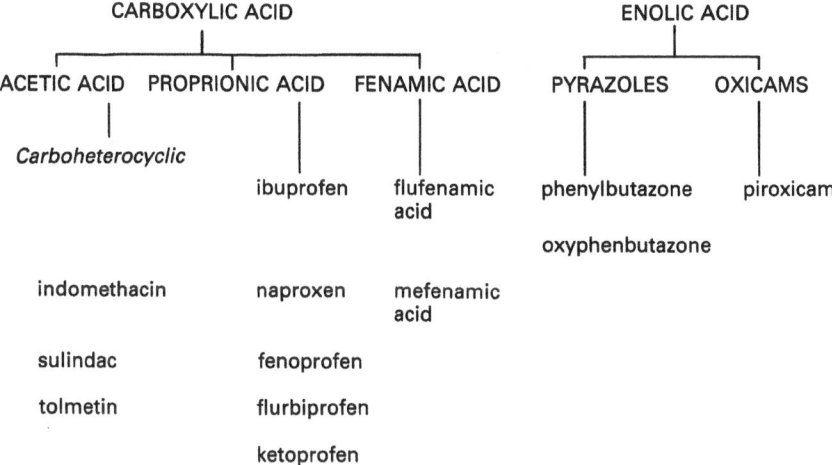

Fig. 1.5. The non-steroidal anti-inflammatory drugs.

GASTROINTESTINAL
INJURY

A variety of gastrointestinal effects, ranging from transient abdominal discomfort to perforation or penetration with a fatal outcome, may be provoked. Gastrointestinal bleeding may range from chronic and occult to acute, massive and life-threatening. Gastric toxicity is linked with the inhibition of prostaglandin synthesis.

The true incidence of aspirin-induced gastrointestinal bleeding is difficult to assess. Loss of blood is commonly occult, and aspirin may be an unrecognised cause of iron-deficiency anaemia. Such bleeding may occur with as little as 50 mg of aspirin daily. Daily doses of 1.5–3 g may provoke blood loss of 3–6 ml, but some patients may lose more than 10 ml daily.

Overt bleeding may develop within a day or two of consumption of aspirin. In the absence of peptic ulceration, bleeding from aspirin is usually associated with erosive gastritis. Bleeding disorders and consumption of alcohol may be predisposing factors. Aspirin is particularly likely to cause acute gastrointestinal haemorrhage in patients with chronic renal failure.

Heavy consumption of aspirin is a recognised aetiological factor in chronic gastric ulcers, characteristically found on the lesser curvature. Unnecessary gastrectomy may be performed because of fear of malignancy.

Although NSAIAs cause less gastrointestinal side-effects than salicylates, none are free of these.

SENSITIVITY REACTIONS

Acute sensitivity responses to aspirin and the NSAIAs are well documented, and cross-sensitivities between aspirin, indomethacin, mefenamic acid, flufenamic acid, phenylbutazone, fenoprofen and ibuprofen, and food additives and colouring agents such as benzoic acid and the acidic yellow dye, tartrazine, have been documented.

Bronchial asthma is an important manifestation of aspirin intolerance. There is an association with urticaria, rhinitis and polyps (the acetylsalicylic acid triad). As little as 30 mg of aspirin may provoke an attack of asthma, which in some cases may progress to anaphylactic shock. The asthma is usually chronic, resistant to treatment and steroid-dependent. Individuals with a positive family history of asthma are prone. Bronchospasm may develop within minutes of aspirin ingestion, sometimes with malaise, angioneurotic oedema, generalised erythema, lacrimation, rhinorrhoea, laryngeal oedema and eosinophilia. Symptoms may persist after aspirin is discontinued.

Vasomotor rhinitis in aspirin-intolerant patients presents as intermittent, profuse, watery nasal secretions, which may be followed by chronic nasal blockade. The mucous membranes of paranasal sinuses show evidence of oedema, and hyperplastic sinusitis may develop. Nasal symptoms generally precede the development of bronchial asthma.

In patients who are hypersensitive to aspirin and

related drugs, repeat administration may result in a severe reaction. Warning signs are a previous history of hypersensitivity reactions to chemicals or drugs, of asthma and nasal polyps.

ANALGESIC NEPHROPATHY

Chronic renal damage may develop as a result of excessive and prolonged use of non-steroidal anti-inflammatory agents. The initial lesions involve renal papillae and inner cortex; the process may extend and in advanced stages necrosis and cavity formation within the medulla may be found. Entire papillae may detach, causing obstruction to urinary flow. Pathological changes develop eventually throughout the kidney.

Ingestion need not necessarily be excessive; renal damage may develop insidiously with regular, long-term usage, especially if fluid intake is low. Combinations of the NSAIAs accentuate the risk. Polycomponent analgesics are often abused; it is not surprising when one considers their psychoactive constituents such as codeine, propoxyphene, meprobamate, barbiturates, antihistamines and caffeine.

The clinical picture may be elusive until advanced damage has developed. The patient may be a dependent personality who smokes and drinks, overrelies on psychotropic agents, may not even provide a history of pain, may not provide a reliable history of drug usage, and is more commonly female. Renal disease is often uncovered in investigation of complaints such as fatigue, anaemia, weight loss, hypertension, peptic ulcer or headache.

REDISTRIBUTIONAL DRUG INTERACTIONS

Aspirin and other NSAIAs may interact with various other medicines, altering their pharmacokinetics by displacement from binding sites on plasma proteins. This applies particularly to the oral anticoagulants, oral hypoglycaemic agents, and barbiturates which bind extensively to plasma albumin. The interaction of NSAIAs with anticoagulants may be serious. A small alteration in concentration of unbound anticoagulant (Fig. 1.6) may substantially increase its potential toxicity.

It is their acidic nature and their propensity for binding to the plasma proteins that these drugs have in common, and displacement from binding sites by another drug in the group is determined by relative affinities.

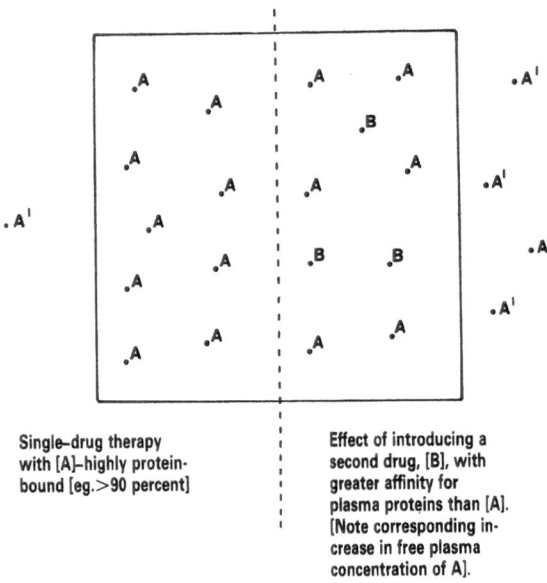

Single–drug therapy with [A]–highly protein-bound [eg.>90 percent]

Effect of introducing a second drug, [B], with greater affinity for plasma proteins than [A]. [Note corresponding increase in free plasma concentration of A].

Fig. 1.6. Redistributional drug interactions. *A*, protein-bound form of drug (A); *A¹*, free plasma form of drug (A)—pharmacologically active; *B*, protein-bound form of drug (B).

GENERAL
CONSIDERATIONS FOR
USE IN CHRONIC
RHEUMATIC
CONDITIONS

i) Considerable inter-individual variation in responses to the anti-inflammatory and analgesic actions and in toxic effects are recognised; the ideal agent and its optimum dose have to be sought in each case.

ii) The therapeutic efficacy of a drug should be evident within 2 weeks. There is little point in prolonging therapy that has not produced a rapid effect.

iii) The significant placebo effect in rheumatic disorders and the variable natural history of the rheumatic diseases are relevant in evaluating response.

iv) There is no evidence that two non-steroidal anti-inflammatory agents used together are more effective than one.

v) Anxiety and depression are frequently associated with chronic pain. Judicious use of psychotropic agents may be valuable.

vi) These agents have effects on the symptomatic aspects of the disease only. The remittive agents (gold, penicillamine, chloroquine and levamisole) modify the natural history of rheumatoid arthritis.

vii) In the event of primary or secondary failure of response the following factors should be reviewed:

a) Lack of compliance
b) Concomitant anxiety or depression
c) Loneliness
d) Coexistent systemic disease
e) Adverse effects of the drugs
f) The quality of overall medical care being offered the patient.

viii) Blood loss due to aspirin can be reduced but not prevented by buffered, effervescent, slow-release and enteric-coated preparations of aspirin. Gastric mucosal damage seems to be less with buffered than with unbuffered aspirin, but buffered aspirin does not reduce the incidence of subjective gastric effects. The non-aspirin NSAIAs are less likely to cause gastrointestinal bleeding than the salicylates.

ix) There are several guidelines for the prevention of analgesic nephropathy:

a) Psychotropic agents should be prescribed separately from analgesic agents, and not in combination formulations.
b) Analgesic prescribing should be critically reviewed at regular intervals.
c) Non-steroidal anti-inflammatory agents should be taken with plenty of water.
d) Special caution should be exercised in patients with impaired renal function.
e) The insidious nature of the development of this nephropathy should be borne in mind.

x) These agents may interact adversely with other drugs that have high affinity for plasma protein binding sites, such as the oral anticoagulants and barbiturates (see redistributional drug interactions, p. 27).

FURTHER READING

Prescott LF (1982) Analgesic nephropathy. Drugs 23:75
Vanecek J (1980) Antipyretic analgesics. In: Dukes MNG (ed) Meyler's side effects of drugs, 9th
    edn. Excerpta Medica, Amsterdam, p 123

1.8 Digitalis

Digitalis glycosides have a narrow therapeutic range, which becomes more restricted with advancing age and severe heart disease. Adjustment of dosage to body weight, renal function (Table 1.7) and clinical factors (Table 1.8) reduces the risk of toxicity, but unpredictable inter-individual variation in response remains.

Blood determinations of digoxin may be of assistance in planning dosage schedules and in identifying toxicity, but digoxin toxicity may occur despite blood levels in the normal range (1.0–2.5 ng/ml), particularly when there is hypokalaemia.

Newborn babies have a resistance to the cardiac effects and toxicity of the digitalis glycosides.

Table 1.7. Adjustment of digoxin dosage to creatinine clearance (Opie 1980)

Creatinine clearance	Approximate digoxin dose
0–25 ml/min	0.125 mg/day
26–49 ml/min	0.1875 mg/day
50–79 ml/min	0.25 mg/day

Table 1.8. Clinical factors altering digitalis sensitivity (based on Opie 1980)

Renal failure (reduced excretion)
Chronic pulmonary disease (hypoxia, acid-base changes)
Hypoxaemia
Hypokalaemia (probable increased binding to the heart)
Hypomagnesaemia (sensitises to toxic effects)
Hypercalcaemia (increases sensitivity to digitalis)

CLINICAL SIGNS OF
DIGITALIS TOXICITY

The gastrointestinal tract, heart and central nervous system may be affected independently or together. Gastrointestinal symptoms are the most common, but they are not necessarily a feature in digitalis toxicity.

Anorexia, nausea and vomiting are mediated in part by chemoreceptors in the area postrema of the medulla rather than by a direct irritant effect of the drug on the gastrointestinal tract. Diarrhoea, abdominal pain and constipation are uncommon.

Tachyarrhythmias or bradyarrhythmias, atrial or ventricular extrasystoles and atrioventricular conduction disturbances may be seen. No particular dysrhythmia is pathognomonic, but in a patient at risk multifocal or paired ventricular extrasystoles (pulsus bigeminus) or paroxysmal atrial tachycardia with varying heart block are strongly suggestive (see Fig. 1.7).

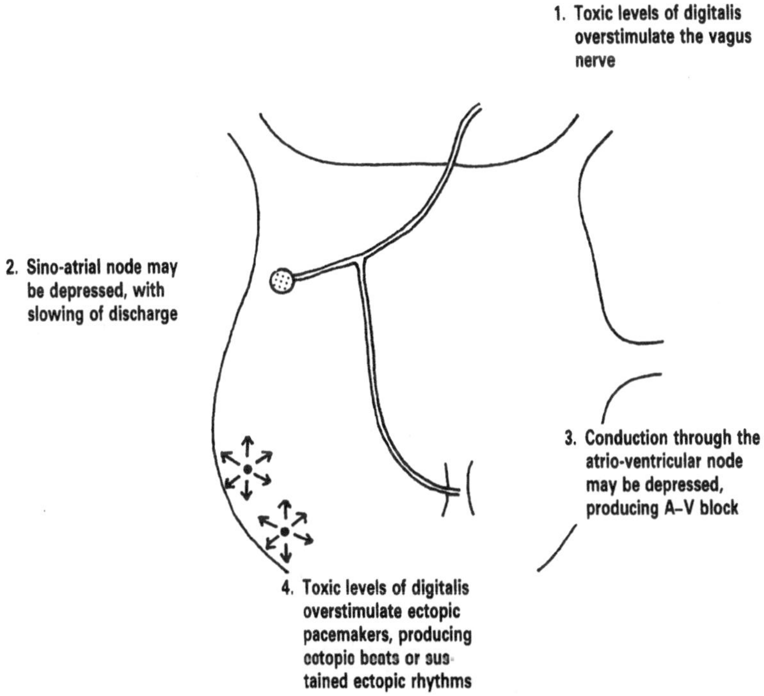

1. Toxic levels of digitalis overstimulate the vagus nerve

2. Sino-atrial node may be depressed, with slowing of discharge

3. Conduction through the atrio-ventricular node may be depressed, producing A-V block

4. Toxic levels of digitalis overstimulate ectopic pacemakers, producing ectopic beats or sustained ectopic rhythms

Fig. 1.7. Toxic effects of digitalis on the heart [reproduced with kind permission from Phibbs B (1978) The cardiac arrhythmias, 3rd edn. Mosby, St Louis].

A life-threatening arrhythmia is more likely to develop when the heart is seriously diseased. Digitalis toxicity may aggravate congestive cardiac failure.

Headache, fatigue, insomnia, malaise, confusion, depression and vertigo are common, and disturbance of colour vision (usually green or yellow) and blurring of vision are well recognised. Convulsions, paraesthesiae, delirium and psychosis are unusual.

EARLY RECOGNITION OF CARDIOTOXICITY

In patients at special risk the following are suggestive signs of cardiotoxicity:
  i) Ectopic impulses, isolated or in runs; slowing of the heart rate;
  ii) Atrioventricular block (the development of first-degree block is suggestive); and
  iii) The association of ectopic ventricular beats with slowed atrioventricular conduction.

The majority of carefully documented patients who have died of digitalis poisoning have developed a cardiac arrhythmia before death.

CONTRAINDICATIONS TO DIGITALIS THERAPY

Heart block may be worsened by digitalis; even first-degree block demands caution, particularly when this is unstable, as in acute myocardial infarction or rheumatic carditis.

In hypertrophic obstructive cardiomyopathy the inotropic effect of digitalis may worsen outflow obstruction. Cautious administration may be necessary when there is coexistent atrial fibrillation and cardiac failure.

The Wolff-Parkinson-White syndrome may be aggravated by digitalis, as anterograde conduction may be further accelerated, with the danger of precipitating ventricular tachycardia.

Digitalis is best avoided in patients about to undergo cardioversion by direct current shock as serious arrhythmias are likely to develop.

MASSIVE DIGITALIS INTOXICATION

This has been reported after accidental and intentional poisoning. The effects in patients with normal hearts are different to those in patients with heart disease. The commonest features have been disturbances in rhythm and atrioventricular conduction, extreme fatigue, severe visual aberrations and transient psychosis. The ophthalmological effects may be due to a transient retrobulbar neuritis. Plasma digoxin levels may be markedly elevated (4–8 times normal), and a well-documented biochemical feature is hyperkalaemia, possibly due to poisoning of ATP-ase systems in the body.

DIGOXIN AND QUINIDINE

Quinidine causes an unpredictably large increase in plasma digoxin and this effect is thought to be due in part to a redistribution of digoxin in the body and a decrease in clearance of digoxin. The relative contributions of redistribution and interference with clearance to the increase in digoxin levels are unknown. Toxicity may result. A patient taking digoxin is advised to reduce the dose by half. Other antiarrhythmic agents such as procainamide, disopyramide and mexiletine do not appear significantly to alter digoxin serum levels, and other forms of digitalis do not interact with quinidine in the same manner.

Further Reading

Beller GA et al. (1971) Digitalis intoxication. N Engl J Med 184:989
Dahlqvist R et al. (1980) Quinidine-digoxin interaction. Br J Clin Pharmacol 9:413
Lely AH, Van Enter CHJ (1970) Large-scale digitoxin intoxication. Br Med J 3:737
Lely AH, Van Enter CHJ (1972) Non-cardiac symptoms of digitalis intoxication. Am Heart J 83:149
Opie LH (1980) Drugs and the heart. Lancet, London

1.9 Sympathomimetic Drugs (See Fig. 1.8)

Most sympathomimetic drugs, however specific to a particular receptor type they are designed to be, will on occasion stimulate central nervous system and cardiovascular functions, resulting in nervousness, insomnia, tremors, dizziness or headache, and palpitations, hypertension and disorders of cardiac rhythm. Sensitivity to the effects of sympathomimetic agents varies markedly from one individual to another. The likelihood of toxic effects is increased when other drugs stimulating the same organs are given at the same time.

ADRENALINE — Modest tachycardia, palpitations, extra-systoles and a rise in blood pressure develop when the limits of tolerance are approached. In sensitive individuals, or with high doses, ventricular fibrillation, pulmonary oedema and severe hypertension may occur. Patients with thyrotoxicosis, angina pectoris, and other forms of heart disease, and those undergoing halothane anaesthesia (which may sensitise the heart to the risk of adrenaline toxicity) are at special risk. Metabolic effects are unlikely because of the short-duration of action of adrenaline.

EPHEDRINE — Systemic effects of ephedrine may be experienced

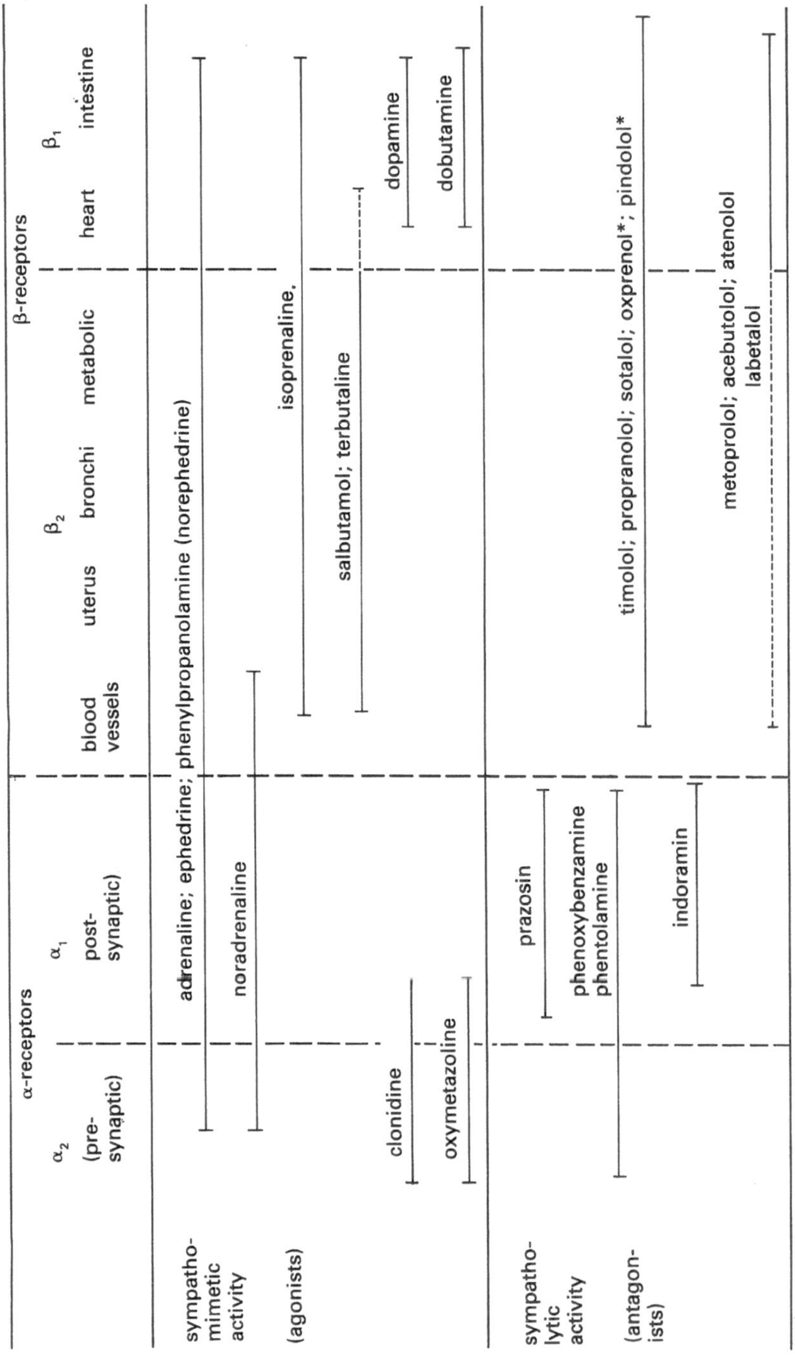

Fig. 1.8. Sympathomimetic and sympathicolytic agents. The *asterisk* signifies intrinsic sympathomimetic (partial agonist) activity. [Based on Lees GM (1981) A hitch-hiker's guide to the galaxy of adrenoreceptors. Br Med J 283:173]

even in the doses normally used in nasal sprays and drops, and in cough or asthma preparations. Ephedrine is longer-acting than adrenaline. It has less effect on the cardiovascular system and a greater effect on the central nervous system. The special risk situations are the same as for adrenaline.

PHENYLPROPANOLAMINE

Phenylpropanolamine is used in mixtures given orally as nasal decongestants and as an anorexiant. It can cause restlessness, anxiety, insomnia, tremor, hypertension and cardiac dysrhythmias. The effects of antihypertensive therapy may be counteracted.

A serious drug-drug interaction, with hypertension and marked reduction of blood supply to the kidneys, spleen, skin and lungs (primary resistance vessels) may occur when α-adrenergic agonists such as phenylpropanolamine and phenylephrine are given together with β-adrenergic blocking agents such as propranolol, which reduce antagonistic vasodilator activity of the same vessels (see Fig. 1.9).

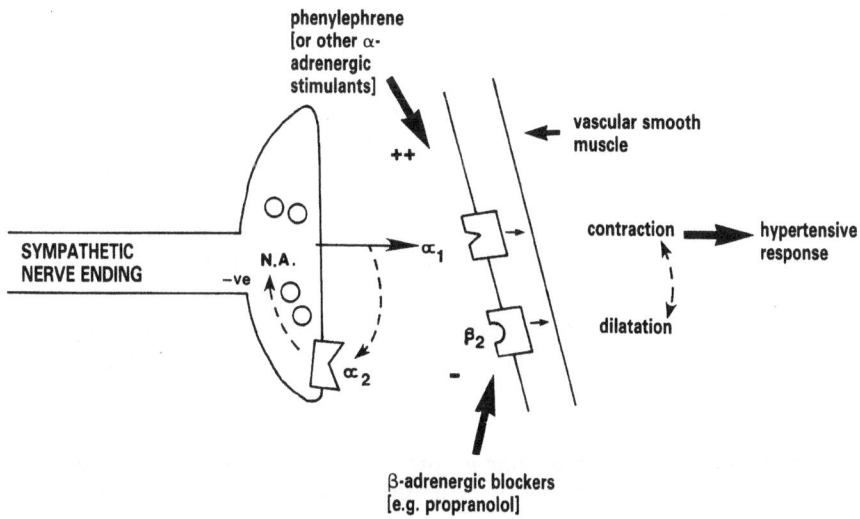

Fig. 1.9. Potential adverse interaction between α-adrenergic agonists and ß-receptor blocking agents, with hypertensive response. N.A., noradrenaline; α, alpha-receptors; ß₂, beta₂-receptors.

NORADRENALINE

Adverse reactions to noradrenaline are mainly adrenergic, involving the central nervous system and small blood vessels. There is little stimulant effect on the β-receptors of the heart, but the rate may be slowed as a reflex response to a rise in blood pressure.

ISOPRENALINE

Isoprenaline is a non-selective β_2-receptor stimulant, widely used in respiratory diseases for relaxation of bronchial smooth muscle. Headache, tremor, apprehension, dizziness, faintness, tachycardia, arrhythmias, palpitations, and induction or aggravation of anginal pain are commonly experienced with isoprenaline. Ventricular fibrillation and cardiac muscle necrosis have resulted when isoprenaline has not been administered with caution. Relaxation of bronchial smooth muscle may adversely affect the ventilation-perfusion ratio, aggravating hypoxaemia at the same time that it diminishes airway resistance. Paradoxical bronchospasm may occur.

BETA$_2$-
SELECTIVE AGENTS

β_2-Selective agents such as salbutamol and terbutaline which are used in the treatment of bronchospasm and for the arrest of premature labour are not free of cardiac effects. Tremor, agitation, tachycardia and cardiac arrhythmias may occur in sensitive individuals. Approximately one individual in ten will experience tachycardia with therapeutic doses. Risk situations are as for other sympathomimetic agents. With repeated administration resistance may develop to the bronchodilator effect.

Administration in nebulised form has produced a minimum of adverse effects, probably because of the fine adjustment of dose with this approach.

These drugs may have adverse metabolic effects in the diabetic patient. Severe hypoglycaemia and keto-acidosis have been described.

DOPAMINE AND
DOBUTAMINE

Dopamine is converted in the body to noradrenaline. It is a natural catecholamine and central nervous system transmitter used therapeutically in shock and heart failure. Ectopic beats, tachycardia, palpitations, anginal pain, bradycardia, acceleration of cardiac conduction, and a rise or fall in blood pressure may result from its use in these situations. Peripheral vascular ischaemia and gangrene are a danger in patients with impaired circulation due to arteriosclerosis, diabetes mellitus, or Raynaud's disease. Angina pectoris may be precipitated.

Dobutamine is a relatively selective β_1-agonist, with only slight β_2-and α-receptor activity. Its positive inotropic action is achieved with less vasoconstrictive effects than with dopamine. An increase in heart rate occurs routinely, and occasionally marked tachycardia is induced.

CLONIDINE

Clonidine has central nervous and peripheral α-adrenergic stimulating actions, and it also suppresses plasma renin activity. Its imidazolidine structure is similar to naphazoline and oxymetazoline, which are used as nasal decongestants. Drowsiness, lethargy, depressed sensorium and, in some patients, respiratory depression and miosis may develop, simulating narcotic overdose.

An initial hypertensive response to clonidine is well recognised, being due to peripheral vasoconstriction. The subsequent antihypertensive effect is thought to be mediated through activation of post-synaptic α-adrenergic receptors in the medulla oblongata that modulate cardiovascular function, producing a decrease in sympathetic efferent stimulation to the heart, kidney and peripheral vasculature, with a resultant fall in blood pressure. (Predominance of the peripheral effect raises the blood pressure, and of the central effect lowers it.) Rebound hypertension after abrupt discontinuation of long-term clonidine therapy is well recognised.

1.10 Alpha-Adrenoreceptor Blocking Agents

The most disabling adverse effect of α-adrenergic blockade is postural hypotension, which is likely to be associated with faintness, dizziness, palpitations and syncopy. Other troublesome adverse effects are lethargy, sedation, depression, impotence, fluid retention and diarrhoea.

Impotence and failure of ejaculation are complications of therapy that may occur even with modest doses. α-Adrenoreceptor activity is required for delivery of semen to the urethra from the vas deferens, seminal vesicles and prostate gland, and also for stimulation of the internal urinary sphincter, preventing retrograde ejaculation. Blockade of α-adrenoreceptors may inhibit these functions, abolishing sexual emission without disturbing erection or the sensation of orgasm (the experience of "dry sex").

PHENOXYBENZAMINE

The pharmacological effects of phenoxybenzamine may be delayed after intravenous administration. Adverse effects characteristic of α-adrenoreceptor blocking agents are seen in a high proportion of patients. Hypotension, syncopy and tachycardia may be disabling. The drug should be used with great caution in patients with cardiovascular disease. Phenoxybenzamine is mainly excreted by the kidney, and dosage should be reduced in renal failure. Long-term use seems to diminish sensitivity of α-adrenergic receptors.

PRAZOSIN

Prazosin is widely used for the treatment of hypertension, and for after-load and pre-load reduction in congestive cardiac failure. It has a toxicity profile similar to the other α-adrenoreceptor blockers.

An important complication is the "first dose phenomenon"—an acute postural hypotensive reaction characterised by faintness, dizziness, palpitations and, occasionally, syncopy. This may follow the initial dose, or it may be a response to subsequent dosage increments. An abrupt loss of sympathetic tone resulting in rapid induction of venous and arteriolar dilatation by a drug with little affinity for the pre-synaptic α_2-receptor may account for the effect. In general, postural hypotension with prazosin is dose-related, exaggerated by exercise, and aggravated by pre-existing sodium restriction or diuretic-induced sodium depletion.

INDORAMIN

Indoramin has a direct cardiac depressant action. Its negative inotropic effect may exacerbate heart failure in patients with cardiac disease. As an antihypertensive its blood pressure lowering effect is not associated with orthostatic hypotension or tachycardia.

1.11 Beta-Adrenoreceptor Blocking Agents

The currently available β-adrenoreceptor blocking drugs share a common safety profile. Adverse reactions are predictable from their pharmacological effects. The most important of these are:

1. *Bradycardia and progressive atrioventricular conduction delay.* In patients with diminished cardiac reserve or congestive cardiac failure, bradycardia and reduction of sympathetic drive may worsen the situation. In second- or third-degree heart block, β-blockers may increase the block and are regarded as contraindicated. These adverse effects are likely to develop irrespective of whether or not the β-blocker is cardioselective, although they are less likely if it is. Patients may rarely be extremely sensitive to the depressant effects of β-adrenoreceptor blockade on the heart. In untreated congestive heart failure the use of β-adrenoreceptor blocking drugs is dangerous; even in hypertensive and thyrotoxic heart failure, where β-blockade might be considered appropriate for treatment of the underlying cause, serious problems of decompensation and even death have developed. Initial conventional digitalis and diuretic therapy in such patients, before they are given β-blockers if these are required, is deemed necessary.

2. *Bronchospasm.* β-Blockade may cause or aggravate bronchospasm, and some individuals may be exquisitely sensitive to this effect. Even those β-blocking agents which are relatively cardioselective may do this when large doses are given. Great caution is necessary in patients with chronic obstructive airways disease and chronic bronchitis. β-Blockers are contraindicated in asthmatic patients or in patients with a history of bronchial asthma. If there is compelling requirement for a β-blocker, this should be initiated under close supervision, with very small doses of a selective β_1-agent in conjunction with topical aerosol administration of a selective bronchodilator such as salbutamol or terbutaline.

3. Treatment with β-adrenoreceptor blockers may cause exacerbation of the symptoms of *peripheral vascular disease* or *Raynaud's phenomenon.* This appears to be due to unopposed arteriolar α-tone, and in patients with ischaemic heart disease further reduction of cardiac output may contribute to the effect. Severe peripheral vascular disease and even gangrene may be precipitated. Demonstration of a clear association between deterioration in the natural history of peripheral vascular disease and the use of β-adrenoreceptor blocking agents has not been demonstrated.

4. A variety of *neuropsychiatric and aesthenic syndromes,* ranging from lassitude when strenuous activity is taken, fatigue, malaise, sleeplessness, vivid dreams and nightmares to overt psychosis, have been reported in association with β-adrenoreceptor blockers. These symptoms may only be elicited on careful questioning. A minority of patients is affected, and sometimes symptoms are overcome by adjustment of dose. Cardioselective and nonselective drugs do not differ in these effects, and there is little evidence that any β-blocker may be superior to any other in this regard. However, a

change to a different agent may lead to a striking improvement based, no doubt, on individual differences in response and perhaps in some cases on a placebo effect.

5. *Severe angina pectoris and fatal cardiac arrhythmias* have occurred when β-adrenoreceptor blocker therapy has been abruptly withdrawn after prolonged use. This may be related to the result of sudden re-institution of sympathetic drive to the myocardium, although factors such as a thrombotic tendency and changes in platelet aggregation may contribute to the effect. Gradual reduction in the dose of the β-blocker rather than abrupt withdrawal will minimise the hazard.

6. The catecholamine response to *hypoglycaemia* resulting in tachycardia and palpitations is inhibited by all β-blockers, but sweating may be increased. Patients need to be made aware that these responses may be masked. β_1-selective agents appear to have an advantage in causing less of a hypertensive reaction to hypoglycaemia in patients coincidentally receiving β-blocking agents (due to unopposed α-activity of the catecholamines released endogenously). (See also p. 120.)

FURTHER READING

Carruthers SG (1980) Anti-anginal and beta-adrenoreceptor blocking drugs. In: Dukes MNG (ed) Meyler's side effects of drugs, 9th edn. Excerpta Medica, Amsterdam, p 295
Day M (1979) Autonomic pharmacology. Churchill Livingstone, Edinburgh
Editorial (1980) Fatigue and beta-blockers. Lancet I:1285
Geyskes GG et al. (1979) Clonidine withdrawal. Br J Clin Pharm 7:55
Lees GM (1981) Clinical guide to adrenoreceptors. Br Med J 183:173
Review (1980) Beta-blockers. Drug Ther Bull 18:61

1.12 Potassium Supplements

Potassium supplementation is frequently prescribed on the assumption that diuretic therapy consistently depletes the total body potassium, and that such depletion is effectively reversed by the doses of potassium that are prescribed. Neither is necessarily the case. Although most diuretics (the potassium-sparing agents excepted) frequently produce a fall in serum potassium, particularly in the early stages of treatment, there is usually little correlation between this and intracellular potassium. Consequently, routine prophylaxis with potassium in patients receiving diuretics is seldom necessary. It is widely believed that the high-ceiling loop diuretics such as frusemide and ethacrynic acid produce a greater fall in serum and intracellular potassium than thiazides. In fact, for an equivalent diuretic effect the opposite is true, and this is reflected in a lower incidence of hypokalaemia in patients on long-term treatment with the former. For supplementation to be effective in a patient who is indeed depleted of potassium, a minimum of 24 mmol will be required daily, and greater amounts may be necessary. Combined diuretic-potassium medications do not normally contain more than 7–8 mmol per unit dosage, which is too little for patients at risk.

Since the plasma potassium forms only 2% of the total body potassium, there is little evidence to suggest that total body depletion occurs until the plasma concentration falls below 2.5–3.0 mmol per litre. Diuretics are likely to reduce serum potassium by 5–10%, and the total body potassium by approximately 20 mmol. This does not represent a hazard except in patients at special risk, such as those with advanced liver disease, secondary hyperaldosteronism associated with renovascular hypertension, nephrotic syndrome, or severe congestive cardiac failure, and patients treated with cardiac glycosides, corticosteroids, or carbenoxolone, which has a potassium-losing effect. The majority who receive diuretics for hypertension or heart failure do not require routine potassium replacement. Loss of potassium may be minimised by a moderate reduction of salt intake to 70–80 mmol daily. This may make it possible for a lower dose of diuretic to be given, as sodium-potassium exchange with potassium loss is likely to be reduced in the distal renal tubule. As a general rule, patients receiving diuretics whose serum potassium falls below 3.5–3.0 mEq/l and who develop symptoms or electrocardiographic signs of hypokalaemia, or asymptomatic patients with a serum potassium of 2.5 mEq/l or less should be given potassium in appropriate dosage.

Potassium supplementation given together with a potassium-sparing diuretic such as spironolactone or triamterene (a regimen which is not infrequently prescribed) may produce a potentially dangerous hyperkalaemia. This situation represents one of the most commonly recognised causes of drug-related mortality. The danger is greatest in patients in renal failure who cannot eliminate excess potassium adequately.

FURTHER READING

Anonymous (1978) Combination of a diuretic with potassium. Drug Ther Bull 16:73
Beeley L (1980) Potassium replacement with diuretics. Adverse Drug Reaction Bull No 84, 304
Beeley L (1980) Potassium supplements. J. R. Coll Physicians Lond 14:58
Henschke PJ et al. (1981) Diuretics and the institutional elderly. J Am Geriatr Soc 29:145

1.13 Nitrates

Nitrates are first-line therapy in angina pectoris. They cause venous dilatation by a primary effect on capacitance vessels; the resultant blood pooling reduces pre-load on the heart, which in turn relieves ventricular work. Nitrates have a lesser effect on arterioles, and they do not appreciably alter the calibre of atherosclerotic coronary arteries. In these actions nitrates are not consistently effective, and the appropriate dose has to be found for each individual.

In the treatment of heart failure nitrates are useful when pulmonary wedge pressure is elevated, and in acute pulmonary oedema and pulmonary congestion they may confer a "pharmacological phlebotomy". In severe failure they may be useful in combination with prazosin or hydralazine. Because of their modest and inconsistent effect on arterioles nitrates are not suitable for the management of hypertension.

ADVERSE EFFECTS   The most troublesome and frequently dose-limiting side-effect of the nitrates is headache, which tends to lessen with continued use. Idiosyncratic severe hypotension with bradycardia may occasionally occur; its mechanism seems to be more complex than a vasodilator effect. A simple hypotensive effect may be experienced by sensitive individuals; this is unusual in patients with heart failure, but may limit therapy in angina pectoris.

A modest reduction in arterial oxygen saturation attributable to nitrates is explicable on grounds of a ventilation-perfusion imbalance created as a result of small vessel dilatation in the pulmonary circulation.

TOLERANCE   In munitions workers exposed to nitrates for long periods, acute withdrawal may result in angina pectoris developing, and in such situations myocardial infarction has been described. Although tolerance in patients treated with nitrates long-term has not so far been described, as a general rule it is probably advisable to taper the dosage rather than to discontinue therapy abruptly.

FURTHER READING

Needleman P, Johnson EM (1980) Nitrates. In: Goodman LS, Gilman AG, Gilman A (eds) The pharmacological basis of therapeutics, 6th edn. Macmillan, New York, p 819

1.14 Calcium Antagonists

Drugs which antagonise the flux of calcium into cells through channels in cell membranes may have two actions: alteration of cardiac rhythm, or vasodilation. Verapamil, nifedipine, prenylamine and perhexilene are thought to work primarily in this manner. (Perhexilene has additional modes of action which include quinidine-like and mild diuretic effects). β-Blockers and local anaesthetics also antagonise calcium transport, but this is not their principal effect.

In theory, any of the calcium antagonists should be effective as anti-arrhythmic, anti-anginal, antihypertensive or anti-cardiac failure agents, but clinical experience with them is limited, and their place in the treatment of these conditions has still to be established.

VERAPAMIL

Verapamil is widely prescribed for supraventricular cardiac arrhythmias, as its principal clinical effect is to increase the refractoriness of the atrioventricular node. When given intravenously to patients with heart block or impaired function of the sinus node (e.g. sick sinus syndrome) verapamil may aggravate heart block, or cause sinus bradycardia or sinus arrest. Normal therapeutic doses are unlikely to have a significant cardiodepressive effect, but in patients with diseased hearts or who are under the influence of β-blockade, the negative inotropic effects of verapamil can be very serious. The combination of verapamil with digitalis is potentially dangerous, and the drug is contraindicated in digitalis toxicity.

When heart failure or conduction block are not present, verapamil may actually improve left ventricular performance, as the benefit of restoring a supraventricular arrhythmia to sinus rhythm or reduction of after-load on the left ventricle may outweigh the negative inotropic effect.

NIFEDIPINE

Nifedipine may be usefully combined with a β-blocking agent in angina pectoris, but care has to be taken that the negative inotropic effect of the two agents used together does not precipitate heart failure. The adverse effects of nifedipine are those of a peripheral vasodilator: flushing, palpitations, headache, dizziness and fluid retention. Nifedipine cannot be given by intravenous infusion as it is light-sensitive.

PERHEXILENE

Perhexilene has anti-anginal and anti-arrhythmic activities; its side-effects, which include dizziness, ataxia, impotence, loss of weight, liver disease similar to alcoholic hepatitis, peripheral neuropathy, raised intracranial pressure, and rare cases of papilloedema and blindness, make it prohibitively toxic as a first-line anti-anginal agent, and it is reserved for refractory cases of angina pectoris.

PRENYLAMINE   Prenylamine is less effective but safer than perhexi-
                            lene in angina pectoris. It may cause facial
                            flushing, dizziness, hypotension and myocardial
                            depression. Small doses should be used in patients
                            who are already receiving β-blockers.

DILTIAZEM   Diltiazem differs from other calcium antagonists
                            in having a significantly more pronounced effect
                            on the atrioventricular node than a negative
                            inotropic effect on the myocardium. It has been
                            used in control of supraventricular tachycardia.

FURTHER READING

Editorial (1981) Calcium antagonists and the heart. Br Med J 282:89
Opie LH (1980) Drugs and the heart. Lancet, London

1.15 Benzodiazepines

The benzodiazepines are effective in short-term relief of anxiety. However,
there is widespread concern that they are over-prescribed and that in view of
the potential hazards connected with their use a more rational approach
should be adopted than is often the case.

Once patients have experienced the quick onset of the anxiety-relieving effects
of the benzodiazepines they may become reluctant to relinquish their use. This
group of drugs induces psychological dependence and there is accumulating
evidence of physical dependence as well, which is usually linked to administration of high doses for lengthy periods of several months. There are reports
suggesting that withdrawal symptoms may occur even after discontinuation
of therapeutic doses.

The benzodiazepines are divided into the long-acting and short-acting groups.
The former have half-lives exceeding 20 h and include diazepam, chlordiazepoxide and nitrazepam. The short-acting group includes oxazepam and
temazepam, which have half-lives of less than 10 h. Long-acting benzodiazepines may produce prolonged sedation and, if taken at night-time, remain
active well into the next day. The resultant "hangover" effect may be undesirable and dangerous with regard to driving, climbing heights and operation of
machinery (see section on drugs and driving ability, p. 149). Such risks are
greatly increased by concomitant use of ethanol. The long-acting benzodiazepines are broken down by the liver into one or more active metabolites, some
of which have even longer half-lives than the parent compound. There is a
danger of accumulation in patients with renal and/or hepatic disease, and in
the neonate whose mother may have been given a long-acting benzodiazepine
during labour.

In these circumstances it is considered safer to use short-acting preparations. Long-acting benzodiazepines have a place when it is necessary to maintain sedation throughout the day, e.g. in patients with persistent anxiety when once-daily administration (preferably at night) should suffice. It is inadvisable to prescribe one type of benzodiazepine at night and another during the day.

GUIDELINES FOR USE

i) Patients should only be given a benzodiazepine if there is a definite clinical indication. A sleepness night or the anxieties of everyday life are not adequate justification for their prescription where counselling and reassurance may be more appropriate.

ii) The primary indication for a benzodiazepine is anxiety which is pathological or incapacitating.

iii) The use of benzodiazepines for psychosomatic disorders, tension headaches and painful conditions is not recommended, unless anxiety is a predominant feature.

iv) The benzodiazepines have no antipsychotic properties. They have no therapeutic value in cases where anxiety is secondary to an underlying depression (a common occurrence), which may in fact be aggravated by their use.

v) Benzodiazepines should be prescribed for a strictly limited period, as their long-term efficacy has not been established. Particular caution is necessary where patients have personality disorders or a history of alcohol and/or drug abuse.

vi) Benzodiazepines are preferably avoided in children, and during pregnancy and lactation.

vii) When patients are being withdrawn from prolonged treatment such withdrawal must be gradual.

DEPENDENCE

The majority of cases of dependence upon benzodiazepines have occurred after prolonged administration of larger doses than those normally recommended. Most patients reported had taken doses at least twice and often four times those normally prescribed, often concurrently with alcohol or other drugs. (Less than 50% took benzodiazepines alone.)

The clinical manifestations of benzodiazepine abstinence in dependent subjects resemble those seen with sedatives, barbiturates and alcohol. After withdrawal the signs of the abstinence syndrome usually develop between the third and sixth days owing to the long duration of elimination of many of the benzodiazepines. The effects tend to last for a shorter time and are less florid than those seen in the barbiturate-withdrawal state.

The mildest symptoms of benzodiazepine withdrawal are anxiety, apprehension, insomnia, dizziness and anorexia. When the drug has originally been prescribed for an anxiety state, it may be impossible to decide on clinical grounds whether such symptoms reflect withdrawal or a recurrence of the underlying disorder, which is due to premature discontinuation of therapy. Weaning dependent patients from benzodiazepines is likely to be less difficult than when a comparable degree of dependence exists with other drugs.

The manifestations of advanced physical dependence include muscular weakness, tremor, postural hypotension, hyperthermia, convulsions, confusional states and psychosis. The more florid symptoms are rare.

FURTHER READING

Committee on the Review of Medicines (1980) Systematic review of the benzodiazepines. Br Med
    J 281: 910
Folb PI (1980) Benzodiazepine-type dependence. In: The safety of medicines: evaluation and
    prediction. Springer, Berlin Heidelberg New York, p 39

1.16 Tricyclic Antidepressants

CARDIOTOXICITY

The tricyclic antidepressants have a reputation for cardiotoxicity, derived largely from evidence that an overdose can produce marked disturbances in cardiac rhythm and impairment of intraventricular conduction. There have also been reports of unexplained death in depressed patients with other medical illnesses who were receiving amitriptyline, thus raising concern that this group of agents might also be cardiotoxic in patients receiving standard clinical doses.

The tricyclics have several different actions on the heart, which include an atropine-like anticholinergic effect, quinidine-like influences on atrioventricular conduction, blockade of noradrenaline receptors with increased local catecholamine concentration and resultant sympathomimetic activity on rhythm and rate, and a suggested inhibitory effect on contractility of cardiac muscle with reduced cardiac output. In carefully controlled studies it has appeared that depressed patients with heart disease can be given tricyclic antidepressants without danger of major adverse effects on cardiac rhythm or left ventricular pump function, and without undue risk, provided the drugs are administered with care. However, these remarks have to be qualified by the comment that patients with pre-existing severe impairment of myocardial function may be particularly susceptible to the negative inotropic action of the tricyclics, which have not been properly studied in this category of patients.

It has also been suggested that tricyclic antidepressants may contribute to the sudden death sometimes noted in depressed patients. There has been no clear evidence of this and the Boston Collaborative Surveillance Programme found no increase in such deaths in patients with myocardial disease receiving tricyclics. Nevertheless, it is generally accepted that caution is necessary in prescribing this category of medicines in the presence of severe myocardial disease, cardiac arrhythmias, conduction defects, an abnormal electrocardiogram, marked atherosclerosis or other forms of cardiovascular disease.

POSTURAL HYPOTENSION

Postural hypotension is a potential risk of therapeutic doses of the tricyclics. It is quite common and it can be severe and disabling. In patients without underlying cardiovascular disease this is likely to be the only serious adverse effect developing in the cardiovascular system. The problem increases dramatically with age, and with coronary or cerebral insufficiency. Not all the tricyclic antidepressants necessarily carry the same order of risk in this regard. The mechanism involved probably includes α-adrenergic blockade in the peripheral circulation. In most cases it can be effectively handled without interrupting therapy by assuring adequate fluid intake, controlled intake of sodium and potassium and by use of elastic stockings and maintenance of muscle tone in the lower extremities through walking and other exercise. Elevation of the head of the bed at night maintains peripheral vascular tone.

ANTICHOLINERGIC
EFFECTS

The maximum doses that can be given to individual patients are limited most often by anticholinergic side-effects. A marked variability between patients in tolerance to the anticholinergic actions of the tricyclic antidepressants is recognised; this is no doubt related in part to an increased sensitivity (possibly at the receptor level) among older patients, and to considerable variations in blood levels amongst patients receiving comparable doses. Even in the same patient a blood level may vary significantly at different times. As much as tenfold differences in plasma levels between patients receiving equal dosages of the same tricyclic drugs have been documented.

The characteristic effects of cholinergic blockade produced by these agents on the heart and central nervous system are described on p. 175–178. The problems of interference with temperature control, central nervous system depression with impairment of fine motor activity and concentration, interaction with other central nervous system depressants and the potential hazards of delirium, mania and an "anti-cholinergic psychosis", which are noted with anticholinergic agents in general, are applicable to this particular group of medicines.

Peripheral anticholinergic side-effects such as dry mouth, constipation, urinary retention and pupillary dilation with consequent blurring of vision and changes in visual accommodation are well recognised with the tricyclics. Caution has to be exercised in patients with glaucoma or urinary tract obstruction due to prostatic hypertrophy. Not infrequently there is little relation between peripheral evidence of anti-cholinergic activity on the one hand and central nervous system or cardiac anticholinergic effects on the other.

EPILEPSY

The overall incidence of seizures during treatment with the tricyclics is approximately 1%, although this may be lower in patients who do not have a background of epilepsy. Although it is suggested that tricyclic antidepressants predispose to epilepsy, the subject has undergone little systematic study. The factors presumed to predispose to seizures during tricyclic therapy are a history of epilepsy, a convulsive disorder in the family, preexisting abnormalities of the electroencephalogram, postnatal brain damage, head trauma, cerebrovascular disease, recent electroconvulsive therapy and concomitant phenothiazine treatment.

ACUTE WITHDRAWAL
EFFECTS

An acute syndrome has been associated with sudden withdrawal of tricyclics, namely, nausea, vomiting, headache, dizziness, anxiety and irritability, weakness and fatigue, sweating, chills, abdominal cramps, coryza and even central nervous system effects such as delirium. Withdrawal symptoms usually cease within 48 h of therapy being discontinued. There has been a report of a panic-anxiety reaction on amitriptyline withdrawal. As a general principle slow reduction of dosage where therapy is to be discontinued seems advisable, and this is probably of special importance in patients with a cardiac rhythm disorder.

FURTHER READING

Aghawewa MO (1981) Symptoms of withdrawal from tricyclic antidepressants. Can Med Assoc J 125:420
Glassman AH, Bigger JT (1981) Cardiovascular effects of therapeutic doses of tricyclic antidepressants. Arch Gen Psychiatry 38:815
Glassman AH et al. (1979) Imipramine-induced orthostatic hypotension. Lancet I:468
Lowry MR, Dunner FJ (1980) Seizures during tricyclic therapy. Am J Psychiatry 137:11
Rodstein M (1979) Cardiovascular side-effects of long-term therapy with tricyclic antidepressants in the aged. J Am Geriatr Soc 27:231
Veith RC et al. (1982) Cardiovascular effects in depressed patients with chronic heart disease. N Engl J Med 306:954

1.17 Methylphenidate

Many hyperkinetic children are treated with psychostimulants, of which methylphenidate (Ritalin, United Kingdom) is most commonly used. Children who do not have brain damage frequently respond to methylphenidate, becoming less restless and impulsive. They show increased attention, less emotional lability, and increased responsiveness to social reinforcement. It is important that this therapy should be regarded as short-term intervention until more positive social and school behaviour can be established.

Methylphenidate metabolises mainly to ritalinic acid, which has poor lipid solubility, and to other lipid-soluble metabolites which may be pharmacologically active. The drug is a fairly predictable therapeutic agent and there appears to be little individual variation in its pharmocokinetics. The best results are obtained in children of normal intelligence and emotional adjustment whose distractibility and hyperactivity are associated with evidence of perceptual and motor immaturity—so-called minimal brain dysfunction. Children with undoubted brain damage, including those with cerebral palsy, and children with primary emotional disorders respond less well.

The adverse effects of methylphenidate are anorexia and insomnia, mild nausea, depressive episodes, and suppression of weight and growth. The latter is attributable to anorexia, which may be induced by the medication. Height and weight charts should be kept. Various studies have indicated that inhibition of growth is apparent only with higher doses of methylphenidate, and that doses of 20 mg daily and less are not associated with growth retardation during the prepubertal period; little is known of the growth-related effects of treatment extending through puberty. Most side-effects subside with time, after discontinuation of the drug. Drug-free periods or substitution by placebo should be introduced periodically, and the effects of withdrawal of medication assessed on the appropriate behavioural parameters. A drug-free period is advised over weekends and during school holidays. There does not appear to be any special predisposition of hyperactive children treated with methylphenidate to become drug abusers.

FURTHER READING

Leary PM et al. (1979) Clinical experience with methylphenidate. S Afr Med J 55:374
Roche AF et al. (1979) Effects of stimulant medication on growth of hyperkinetic children. Pediatrics 63:847

1.18 Anorectic Agents

The majority of medicines used for weight reduction fall into one of four categories: sympathomimetic amines, diuretics, methylcellulose or other similar laxatives, and phenolphthalein.

Thyroid hormones have no place in the management of obesity, in the absence of hypothyroidism. Methylcellulose, which is used to increase bulk in the stomach, thus producing a feeling of satiety, does not have any special merit in the treatment of obesity. There is no rational basis for the use of laxatives or diuretics in the management of obesity, and their administration may be associated with risks such as electrolyte imbalance. Phenolphthalein is not effective for this purpose.

SYMPATHOMIMETIC
AMINES

The majority of the sympathomimetic amines bear a structural similarity to amphetamine (phenylethylamine moiety). Amphetamines and related compounds act chiefly by stimulating the ventromedial hypothalamic (satiety) centres, but they may also stimulate free fatty acid release by adipose tissue. They are most effectively used after the effects on the hunger satiety pattern of the appropriate reducing diet have been determined. The effective duration of treatment of the sympathomimetic amines is usually 4–6 weeks, after which the weight-losing effect is limited by development of tolerance. There is no evidence that they are of value in the long-term management of obesity.

The amphetamine-related anorexigenic agents are regarded as having a potential for creating dependence, which is related to the dose and duration of their administration. Mazindol and phentermine may have a different action to the other sympathomimetic agents, and less dependence-producing potential. The place of sympathomimetic amines in the management of mild obesity is very limited.

A list of sympathomimetic agents with anorexiant activity, along with their structural formulae, is given in Table 1.9.

SAFETY

Most patients develop effects from sympathomimetic actions of the centrally acting agents: dry mouth, restlessness, irritability, insomnia and sometimes constipation. Cardiac patients are at risk because of adrenergic effects on the heart rate and potentiation of cardiac arrhythmias. In patients with hypertension the beneficial effects of loss of weight may outweigh the risks.

Centrally acting appetite suppressants carry the potential risk of dependence. For most the central stimulant and anorectic effects have proven inseparable. Psychotic reactions, anxiety, agitation, excitability and restlessness may develop. A past history of alcohol or drug abuse, or psychiatric illness, and prolonged administration may increase the chances of dependence.

Sympathomimetic amines are contraindicated in patients being treated with monoamine oxidase inhibitors, ephedrine and other sympathomimetic

Table 1.9. Structural formulae of sympathomimetic amines [based on The Merck Index, 9th edn (1976) Merck and Co, Inc, Rahway, New Jersey]

Amphetamine	$CH_2.CH.CH_3$ $\quad\quad\mid$ $\quad\quad NH_2$
Benzphetamine	CH_3 $\mid$ $CH_2.CH.N.CH_2.C_6H_5$ $\quad\quad\quad\mid$ $\quad\quad\quad CH_3$
Chlorphentermine	$Cl.$ $\quad CH_3$ $\quad\quad\quad\quad\quad\mid$ $\quad CH_2.C.NH_2$ $\quad\quad\quad\quad\quad\mid$ $\quad\quad\quad\quad CH_3$
Diethylpropion	$CO.CH.N.(C_2H_5)_2$ $\quad\quad\mid$ $\quad\quad CH_3$
d-Norpseudoephedrine	NH_2 $\mid$ $HO.CH.CH.CH_3$
Ephedrine	CH_3 $\mid$ $HO.CH.CH.NH.CH_3$
Fenfluramine	CH_3 $\mid$ $CH_2.CH.NH.C_2H_5$ CF_3

Table 1.9 (*continued*)

Mazindol	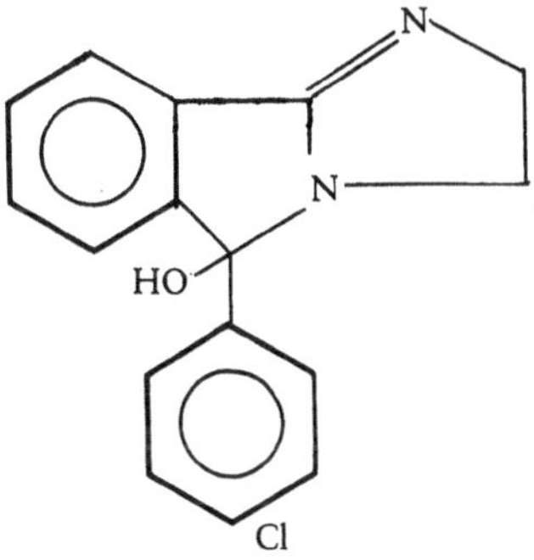

Methamphetamine

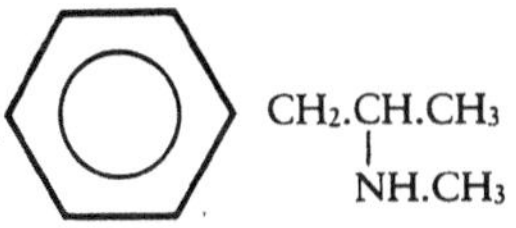

$CH_2.CH.CH_3$
$NH.CH_3$

Phendimetrazine

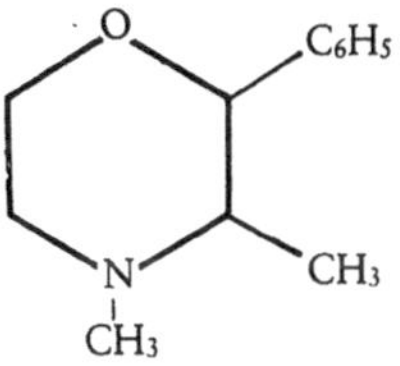

C_6H_5
CH_3
CH_3

Phentermine

CH_3
$CH_2.C.NH_2$
CH_3

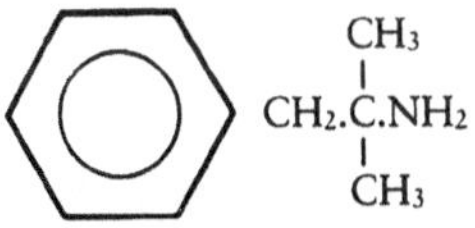

Phenylpropanolamine
hydrochloride
(*dl*-norephedrine
hydrochloride)

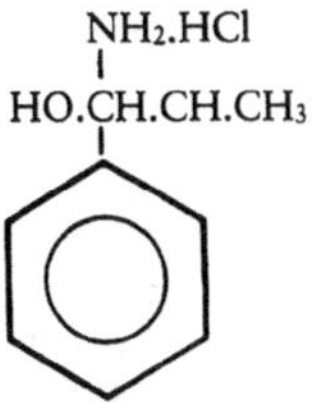

$NH_2.HCl$
$HO.CH.CH.CH_3$

Propylhexedrine

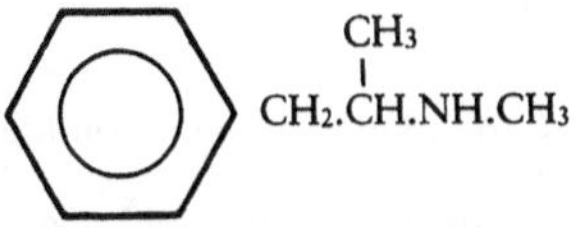

CH_3
$CH_2.CH.NH.CH_3$

agents, as a hypertensive response may result. These drugs should be avoided in children because of the possibility of growth suppression.

FENFLURAMINE

Fenfluramine causes drowsiness in some patients, and in this respect it differs from the other agents of its class. Dependence is rare, but abrupt withdrawal may induce depression. It should be avoided in patients with a history of depression. Its sedative action may be of value in co-existing anxiety states.

PHENYLPROPANOLAMINE

Phenylpropanolamine is freely available in various countries as a slimming aid. Perhaps because of its particularly widespread use, special attention has been focused on its safety. After therapeutic and excessive doses arrhythmias, severe hypertension and myocardial damage have been described. Hypertensive crises may occur when phenylpropanolamine is taken with monoamine oxidase inhibitors, methyldopa, oxprenolol or indomethacin. There have been reports of psychotic reactions, mania and hallucinations. Paranoid reactions and grand mal seizures have also been noted.

COMPARATIVE PHARMACOLOGICAL EFFECTS

The pharmacological properties of various centrally acting agents are presented in Table 1.10.

Table 1.10. Pharmacological effects of certain centrally acting anorectic agents

Drug	Central nervous system stimulation	Peripheral adrenergic activity	Dependence production / tolerance
d-Amphetamine	++++	++	+++
l-Amphetamine	+	+++	+++
Ephedrine	++	++	++
Fenfluramine	–	+	+
Mazindol	+	±	+
Methamphetamine	++++	+ (+++ in large doses)	
Phendimetrazine	++	+	+

FURTHER READING

Committee on Alcoholism and Addiction and Council on Mental Health (1966) Dependence on amphetamines. JAMA 192:193
Nir I (1980) Certain nervous system stimulants and anorectic agents. In: Dukes MNG (ed) Meyler's side effects of drugs, 9th edn. Excerpta Medica, Amsterdam, p 1

Therapeutics Advisory Committee of the Royal Australasian College of Physicians for the Australian Department of Health (1975) Report on anorectic drugs and central nervous stimulants. Aust J Pharm 56:90

1.19 Addition of Drugs to Intravenous Fluids

The drugs added to intravenous (IV) fluids are mainly antibiotics, electrolytes, vitamins and, to a lesser extent, agents such as aminophylline and heparin. The hazards of introducing an additive into an intravenous drip include breakdown of sterility, drug incompatibility, risk of thrombophlebitis, introduction of particulate matter when reconstituted powdered drugs are used and an increased incidence of dose-related and idiosyncratic adverse drug reactions.

A working approach to antibiotic incompatibilities for IV use is suggested in Table 1.11. The drug incompatibilities listed are those which are best documented.

The following proposals for addition of drugs to intravenous fluids are conservative, and aimed at maximum safety:

1. The addition of drugs to IV fluids should be discouraged except in cases of emergency and for the treatment of infants.

2. Where addition of drugs to an IV fluid unit is indicated only one drug should be added.

3. The only IV fluids to be used for this purpose are isotonic saline and 5% dextrose. More complicated electrolyte solutions and other fluids which contain amino acids and emulsions are not suitable for the purpose of adding drugs.

Table 1.11. Intravenous antibiotic admixture incompatibilities[1, 2]

	Amino acids	Aminophylline	Amphotericin B	Ampicillin	Calcium chloride	Carbenicillin	Chloramphenicol	Cimetidine	Erythromycin	Heparin Na+	Hydrocortisone	Methylprednisolone	Sodium bicarbonate	Tetracyclines	Vitamin infusions	Vancomycin
Ampicillin[3,4]								+					+			
Carbenicillin		+					+	+	+				+	+		
Chloramphenicol					+			+	+		+	+	+	+	+	+
Clindamycin								+						+		
Erythromycin[4]						+	+	+		+				+	+	
Methicillin[4]								+			+		+	+	+	
Penicillin[5]	+		+					+		+			+	+	+	+
Tetracyclines[4,6]		+	+	+	+	+	+	+	+	+	+	+			+	

Numbers refer to the following notes

Notes:

1. No antibiotics (or any other drugs) can safely be added to the following:
   blood and blood components (human)
   fat emulsion 10%
   amino acid solutions

2. The following antibiotics are incompatible with all other drugs in admixture:
   cefazolin sodium   lincomycin hydrochloride
   gentamicin   minocycline hydrochloride
   kanamycin sulphate   oxacillin sodium

3. Sodium ampicillin is an alkaline antibiotic, and it may raise the pH of the intravenous fluid to 8.0 or higher, at which level ampicillin is slowly inactivated. In more acid solutions, such as 5% dextrose in water (pH about 4.7), ampicillin is more stable, but the pH of individual bottles may vary. For these reasons it is advisable to avoid adding ampicillin to intravenous solutions whenever possible.

4. The following indicates the stability of some antibiotics in intravenous fluids:

Drug	Intravenous fluid	Percentage of drug activity lost	time (h)
Erythromycin	Dextrose 5%/saline	21	12
Nafcillin Na+	Dextrose 10%	47	24
Oxytetracycline	Dextrose 5%	25	24
Ampicillin	Dextrose 5%	24	8
Methicillin Na+	Dextrose/saline	50	0.5
Methicillin Na+	Dextrose	50	4.6

5. Penicillin G and semisynthetic pencillins are almost completely inactivated within a few hours in carbohydrate solutions containing sufficient bicarbonate to elevate the pH above 8.0. Penicilloic acid, which appears to have a role in some allergic reactions, is a major product of such inactivation.

6. Tetracyclines form stable insoluble chelates with polyvalent metal cations (e.g. Al^{3+}, Ca^{2+}, Fe^{2+}, Mg^{2+}) that may be present in infusion fluids or in other medicines administered simultaneously.

7. Table 1.11 and these notes are based on the following:

Engel G (1971) Addition of drugs to intravenous fluids. Med J Aust 2:962
Newton DW (1978) Physicochemical determinants of incompatibility and instability in injectable drug solutions and admixtures. Am J Hosp Pharm 35:1213
Kucers A, Bennett N McK (1979) The use of antibiotics. Heinemann, London
A Guide to IV Admixture Compatibility (1980) Medical Economics Company, Oradell, New Jersey (by arrangement with New England Deaconess Hospital, Boston, Massachusetts)

The following proposals for addition of drugs to intravenous fluids are conservative, and aimed at maximum safety:

1. The addition of drugs to IV fluids should be discouraged except in cases of emergency and for the treatment of infants.

2. Where addition of drugs to an IV fluid unit is indicated only one drug should be added.

3. The only IV fluids to be used for this purpose are isotonic saline and 5% dextrose. More complicated electrolyte solutions and other fluids which contain amino acids and emulsions are not suitable for the purpose of adding drugs.

1.20 Parenteral Nutrition*

Total intravenous nutrition has proved to be life saving in cases of "intestinal failure", i.e. when the absorptive capacity of the gut is reduced by disease, massive resection, or short-circuiting of large segments of bowel to an extent that the patient cannot maintain weight and nutrition. Certain patients require permanent support in this manner; in most cases parenteral nutrition given during the crisis of a disease allows time for remission, or for the remaining bowel to adapt, thus enabling the patient eventually to return to taking food by mouth.

Scrupulous control in the preparation of intravenous nutritional solutions and monitoring of blood electrolytes, osmolality, glucose, pH and body temperature during administration have contributed considerably to improving their safety. At the same time various problems have emerged as a result of the possibilities that now exist for prolonged therapy.

MICRONUTRIENT
DEFICIENCIES

In patients receiving total parenteral nutrition (TPN) for prolonged periods (months or years) there is increasing risk of the development of deficiency states of trace elements or micronutrient imbalance. Details of micronutrient deficiency syndromes complicating long-term TPN which have been described are given in Table 1.12. In general, the relatively stable patient who receives long-term parenteral nutrition tends to develop more clearly defined syndromes of micronutrient imbalance than the acutely ill hospital patient who often has multiple metabolic disturbances. No definite standards have been established for the additional supply of micronutrients in total parenteral nutrition, and little is understood concerning the pathogenesis of most of these deficiency syndromes.

Table 1.12. Micronutrient deficiency syndromes complicating total parenteral nutrition

Deficiency syndrome	Clinical and biochemical features
Vitamin A deficiency	Night blindness with absence of rod function; decreased cone function resulting in "bleaching" of colours by day. Marked reduction in the normal serum vitamin A levels. Rapid clinical response to vitamin A

*The section on parenteral nutrition is reproduced in part with permission from Folb PI (1982, 1983) Intravenous infusions—solutions and emulsions. In: Dukes MNG (ed) Meyler's side effects of drugs, Annuals 6 and 7. Excerpta Medica, Amsterdam, p 298 and p 337

Table 1.12. *(Continued)*

Deficiency syndrome	Clinical and biochemical features
Zinc deficiency	Progressive, widespread, painful and inflamed skin eruptions with variable redness, scaliness and blistering. Impetigo-like lesions in some areas. The extremities of upper and lower limbs are often affected. There may be rapid loss of hair. A rapid response to zinc or to a normal diet can be anticipated
Selenium deficiency	Muscle pain and tenderness, inhibiting mobility, are usual. Marked reduction in blood Se levels and in 24-h urinary Se excretion, which respond dramatically within a few days to Se supplementation. Gastrointestinal disturbance, tiredness, hair and nail changes, dermatitis, fatty degeneration of the liver and kidney, porphyrinuria, achylia and cardiac disturbances have been described. Factors suggested as influencing Se status of patients receiving TPN include geographical location (low soil content of Se), preceding nutritional state, pre-existing disease, Se content of TPN solutions, infusion of blood and blood substitutes, gastrointestinal losses especially when excessive, trauma, infection, age and duration of TPN
Chromium deficiency	Isolated chromium deficiency in man has not been clearly documented, but there is some evidence that it results in glucose intolerance, neuropathy (ataxia and peripheral nerve conduction defects), high serum free fatty acid levels, low respiratory quotient, and abnormalities of nitrogen metabolism. Chromium and insulin seem to be closely inter-related in several aspects of metabolism
Hypomagnesaemia	Tremor, weakness and irritability are the most usual signs. Patients may have low serum levels of magnesium; symptoms are relieved following magnesium administration. (Because magnesium is primarily intracellular, low serum levels do not necessarily represent a true body deficiency. The most sensitive indicator is a fall in the urinary magnesium concentration)
Iron deficiency	Iron is not generally added to TPN solutions because of concern about physical incompatibility and the risk of anaphylaxis with available iron-dextran preparations. Iron-deficiency anaemia is one of the most common complications of TPN
Choline deficiency	A fall in free plasma choline levels was demonstrated 2 weeks after the start of TPN in one study. An increase in SGOT coincided with the fall in plasma choline but other biochemical indices of liver function did not change significantly
Thiamine deficiency	A small number of patients reported in the literature have died suddenly from acute Wernicke's encephalopathy (WE) following prolonged TPN. A minority demonstrated the classic signs of WE such as ataxia, nystagmus and ophthalmoplegia. The clinical course of the remainder was one of confusion, convulsions and coma
Copper deficiency	Leucopenia, neutropenia, and/or anaemia are characteristic of copper deficiency in patients receiving TPN solutions. A decrease in serum copper is supporting evidence of copper deficiency. Administration of copper promptly corrects the haematological abnormalities

Note: Reference sources to these micronutrient deficiencies are quoted in Folb PI (1982) Intravenous infusions—solutions and emulsions. In: Dukes MNG (ed) Meyler's side effects of drugs, Annual 6. Excerpta Medica, Amsterdam, p 298

METABOLIC BONE
DISEASE

Numerous cases of metabolic bone disease developing in patients on long-term TPN have been reported. The clinical features are of insidious onset of bone pain, which may become severe and cause considerable disability. The pain is predominantly peri-articular and experienced particularly in weight-bearing areas. Urinary calcium excretion and serum alkaline phosphatase levels are invariably raised. Either patchy osteomalacia with reduced mineralisation and decreased bone turnover or a hyperkinetic bone picture, compatible with hyperparathyroidism, may be seen in biopsy specimens.

Symptoms usually resolve 1–2 months after discontinuation of TPN infusions, despite nutritional deterioration in some cases.

The pathogenesis of the bone disease of TPN is not understood, and it may be that there are several reasons for its development, amongst them quantitative changes in the vitamin D content of the parenteral nutrition solution.

HEPATIC DYSFUNCTION

Hepatobiliary dysfunction is a recognised complication of prolonged TPN in infants and children. Although the cause is not understood, certain aspects of its natural history, pathology and aetiology are becoming clear.

Cholestasis appears to be the primary lesion, and direct hyperbilirubinaemia and raised serum bile acids occur prior to hepatocellular necrosis. As a result of prolonged and persistent cholestasis severe hepatocellular damage may develop; the histological changes may mimic extrahepatic biliary atresia and may progress to cirrhosis.

Immature infants are at highest risk and the more immature the neonate, the more severe is the cholestasis. Hepatobiliary dysfunction is common when TPN is administered for longer than 60 days, and the development of cholestasis appears to be closely correlated with the duration of therapy.

In the majority of the comparatively small number of cases reported, clinical and bio-chemical improvement has been noted within 2 weeks of discontinuing parenteral nutrition, and recovery has appeared complete within a matter of months. However, follow-up liver biopsy in several cases has revealed evidence of mild persistent cholestasis and periportal fibrosis. Cholelithiasis is an additional potential complication.

Close minitoring for signs of liver dysfunction in neonates and infants receiving prolonged parenteral nutrition is essential.

FAT OVERLOAD
SYNDROME

Infants of very low birth weight are generally intolerant of conventional doses of Intralipid, and fat embolism is well described in infants after intravenous fat infusions. This therapeutic complication has been termed "fat overloading syndrome" and it bears a clinical similarity to post-traumatic fat embolism. From reported cases it appears that in infants a total daily dose of 4 g lipid/kg body weight should not be exceeded, and in infants of very low birth weight (less than 33 weeks' gestation) a daily dose of 3 g/kg of Intralipid should probably be regarded as a maximum.

It is likely that accumulation of fat in the blood occurs when lipoprotein lipase becomes saturated, as a result of which the fat infusion is faster than it can be cleared by the reticuloendothelial system. Viral infections or heparin administration may impair the metabolism of lipids by peripheral tissues (this effect of heparin may be due to depletion of lipoprotein lipase). Either of these events may tip the balance adversely in a neonate or infant during lipid infusion.

In patients with Intralipid-induced lipaemia pulmonary function studies have revealed decreased pulmonary alveolar membrane diffusion; these changes revert to basal levels when serum lipids are cleared. Neonates with pre-existing pulmonary hypertension may be at greater risk. Pathological findings include histological evidence of pulmonary hypertension, significant lipid filling of the cytoplasm of cells in the arterial wall, lipid deposits in the intima of small muscular arteries which reduce the luminal diameter of the affected vessels, and pulmonary parenchymal infiltration by fat.

FURTHER READING

Benjamin DR (1981) Hepatobiliary dysfunction associated with long-term TPN. Am J Clin Pathol
  76:276
Heyman MB et al. (1981) The fat overload syndrome. Am J Dis Child 135:628
Pereira GR et al. (1981) Hyperalimentation-induced cholestasis. Am J Dis Child 135:842
Shike M et al. (1980) Metabolic bone disease in long-term TPN. Ann Intern Med 92:343

1.21 Topical Corticosteroids

All topical corticosteroids have anti-inflammatory, antipruritic and vasoconstrictive activity. The mechanism of the anti-inflammatory effect is unclear.
There is some evidence to suggest that a correlation exists between vasocon-
strictor potency and therapeutic efficacy in man. Another corticosteroid mechanism, an antimitotic effect, is probably the basis for the effective use of
intralesional corticosteroid injection therapy of hypertrophic scars and keloids.

Topical steroids are of value in inflammatory conditions of the skin, other
than those due to infection. Their special use is in severe eczema. They do
not exert a curative action. They provide relief of symptoms and suppress
signs, and are indicated when other measures have proved ineffective. Skin
disorders responsive to topical corticosteroids are listed in Table 1.13.

Table 1.13. Skin disorders responsive to topical corticosteroids

Disorders generally responsive	Disorders normally less responsive[a]
Atopic dermatitis	Discoid lupus erythematosus
Seborrhoeic dermatitis	Necrobiosis lipoidica
Lichen simplex chronicus (localised	Lichen planus
neurodermatitis)	Alopecia areata
Psoriasis (particularly of the face and body	Hypertrophic scars
folds)	Keloids
Allergic contact dermatitis	Pemphigus
	Granuloma annulare
	Pretibial myxoedema
	Psoriasis of palms, soles, elbows and knees
	Acne cysts

[a]These conditions may require higher concentrations and/or greater potency of corticosteroids, or
application with occlusions, or intralesional therapy.

A partial response may in some cases be due to difficulty in delivering the corticosteroid to the
appropriate site in sufficient concentrations.

POTENCY   Topical steroids fall into four groups with regard
                   to potency (Table 1.14). Efficacy and adverse
                   effects are determined by potency. For all topical
                   steroids a dose-response relationship exists, resul-
                   ting in increasing efficacy and toxicity with higher
                   doses. Several-fold differences in dose can override
                   differences in potency between preparations.

Table 1.14. Potency of various topical corticosteroid preparations

Potency	Corticosteroid preparation	Chloro- and fluoro-substitution	Strength (%)
Very potent	Clobetasol dipropionate	9 α fluoro	0.05
Potent	Beclomethasone dipropionate	9 α chloro	0.025
	Betamethasone-17-valerate	9 α fluoro	0.05–0.1
	Betamethasone dipropionate	9 α fluoro	0.05–0.5
	Betamethasone-17-benzoate	9 α fluoro	0.025
	Diflucortolone valerate	6 α 9 α fluoro	0.1
	Fluocinolone acetonide	6 α 9 α difluoro	0.025
	Fluocinonide		0.05
	Fluocortolone acetonide	6 α fluoro 9 α 11 β chloro	0.025
	Fluoromethalone (ophthalmic)	9 α fluoro	0.1
	Flumethasone pivalate	6 α 9 α difluoro	0.02
	Fluprednylidine 21 acetate	9 α fluoro	0.1
	Halcinonide	9 α fluoro 21 chloro	0.1
	Hydrocortisone-17-butyrate	–	0.1
	Triamcinolone acetonide	9 α fluoro	0.01–0.1
Moderate potency	Clobetasone butyrate	9 α fluoro	0.05
	Desoxymethasone	9 α fluoro	0.05
	Dexamethasone	9 α fluoro	0.04
	Fluocortolone pivalate	6 α fluoro	0.1–0.25
	Fluocortolone hexaonate	6 α fluoro	0.1–0.25
	Prednisolone	–	0.5
Weak	Hydrocortisone	–	0.1–1
	Hydrocortisone acetate	–	0.2–0.5

ACTIVITY

A slow-release pharmacokinetic curve has been noted with many topically applied corticosteroids. Ointment bases tend to give better activity of the steroid than creams, lotions or aerosols. Occlusion with a plastic wrap can enhance skin penetration ten-fold. Fluorination of the steroid molecule usually confers high potency; with few exceptions potent topical corticosteroids are 9-fluor-substituted.

LOCAL TOXICITY

The more potent the steroid and the higher the dose, the greater the local adverse effects. These include:

i) Aggravation of any existing infection.

ii) Atrophic changes in the skin leading to thinning, loss of elasticity, striae atrophicae, dilatation of superficial blood vessels, telangiectasiae and ecchymoses. Such changes are particularly likely to occur in areas with the greatest permeability, such as the face, eyelids, axilla, scrotum and possibly the groin, and least likely on the dorsa of the hands, extensor surfaces of the knees and elbows, and the palms and soles.

iii) Acne at the site of application.

iv) Depigmentation.

It is important that the lowest maintenance dose possible should be used.

Potent corticosteroids applied to the face for long periods may cause rosacea-like eruptions which flare after the steroid is withdrawn. They are likely to clear 1–3 months after discontinuing treatment. The danger is that such reactions may be treated with even stronger steroids, making the disorder worse.

Topical steroids can themselves cause an allergic contact dermatitis. This may be due to impurities in the preparation, or in the vehicle, preservative or lanolin.

SYSTEMIC TOXICITY

Absorption is likely when a potent corticosteroid is applied to wide areas of the body or to damaged skin, or when an occlusive dressing is applied. Depression of the hypothalamic-pituitary-adrenal axis (HPA-axis) may result.

Children absorb proportionally larger amounts of corticosteroids applied locally because of a larger skin surface area to body weight ratio. (Tight-fitting nappies or plastic pants should not be used on a child being treated in the nappy area, as these may, in effect, act as occlusive dressings.) Depression of the HPA-axis in children retards growth and development.

Cushing's syndrome is very infrequent.

Patients undergoing major surgery or other acute stress who have previously experienced extensive topical application of potent corticosteroids should receive replacement therapy to prevent a possible adrenal crisis. The real incidence of the latter is not known; it is presumably very uncommon.

MINIMISING RISKS OF
ADVERSE EFFECTS

i) Ideally, topical steroids should be restricted to short courses only.

ii) In the presence of infection appropriate antimicrobial therapy should be instituted concomitantly. Topical corticosteroids are contraindicated in local herpes simplex, vaccinia or varicella infections (exacerbation or dissemination may result).

iii) In facial dermatoses low-potency preparations in short courses are advised, and particular care has to be taken near the eyes.

iv) Topical steroids should not be used in infants and young children.

v) In severe psoriasis potent steroids may induce a generalised pustular psoriasis during therapy or after withdrawal.

USE IN
OPHTHALMOLOGY

Corticosteroids are used in the eye for diseases of the conjunctiva and cornea and of the anterior segment. Therapeutic concentrations are attained in aqueous humour following installation in the conjunctival cul-de-sac. Subconjunctival injection has an important place in the treatment of scleritis, iridocyclitis and various other inflammatory eye conditions. For disease of the posterior segment of the eye systemic administration is necessary.

Three main dangers exist with local use of corticosteroids in the eye:

i) Corneal ulceration may be aggravated. In the treatment of lacerations and abrasions of the eye it is thought that healing may be delayed.

ii) Glaucoma may develop after a week or more of treatment in certain patients. This has not always been reversible on cessation of treatment. The mechanism is not understood, although it is known to have a genetic basis. Intraocular pressure should be monitored when corticosteroids are applied to the eye for more than a few days.

iii) In patients with conjunctivitis, local steroids may mask evidence of progression of infection. In dendritic keratitis (herpes simplex), irreversible clouding of the cornea may result.

There are no differences between the various steroid preparations for ocular use with respect to these adverse effects.

FURTHER READING

British National Formulary (1981) No 2. British Medical Association and The Pharmaceutical Society of Great Britain, p 289
Editorial (1977) Topical steroids. Lancet II:487
Food and Drug Administration Drug Bulletin (1981) 11(3):1
Haynes RCJ, Murad F (1980) Adrenocorticosteroid hormone etc. In: Gilman AG, Goodman LS, Gilman A (eds) The pharmacological basis of therapeutics, 6th edn. Macmillan, New York, p 1466
Kligman AM, Leyden JJ (1974) Adverse effects of fluorinated steroids applied to the face. JAMA 229:60
Maibach HI, Stoughton RB (1973) Topical corticosteroids. Med Clin North Am 57:1253
Vale J, Cox B (1978) Decongestants, antihistamines and anti-inflammatory compounds. In: Drugs and the eye. Butterworth, London, p 83

1.22 Methylene Blue

Methylene blue has weak bacteriostatic activity, and it has been used topically and in the genitourinary tract as an antiseptic. Although it is relatively ineffective for these purposes, many "kidney and bladder preparations" containing methylene blue are freely available in most countries, often over the counter. The use of methylene blue for bacteriostasis can be regarded as obsolete.

Methylene blue has a retarding effect on crystal formation in vitro, and for this reason it enjoyed popularity at one time as treatment for nephrolithiasis. However, its efficacy in prevention or reduction of crystallisation in the urinary tract is not established, and neither are claims for prophylaxis or treatment of nephrolithiasis or bladder calculus.

USE IN
METHAEMOGLOBINAEMIA

In low concentrations methylene blue or the chemically related thionine are capable of hastening the conversion of methaemoglobin to haemoglobin. Methylene blue is therefore of value in the treatment of drug-induced and idiopathic methaemoglobinaemia. It is poorly absorbed from the gastrointestinal tract, and for severe cases of methaemoglobinaemia it has to be given intravenously. Large oral doses have been given with ascorbic acid for idiopathic methaemoglobinaemia. The dye is not effective in methaemoglobinaemia developing in patients with glucose-6-phosphate dehydrogenase deficiency.

TOXICITY   Haemolytic anaemia may develop following large
                            doses of methylene blue. High concentrations
                            oxidise ferrous iron of reduced haemoglobin to
                            the ferric form, resulting in formation of methaem-
                            oglobin. Shock may result. The blue tinge
                            produced by the compound may be difficult to
                            distinguish from true cyanosis.

                            Nausea, abdominal and chest pain, headache,
                            dizziness, mental confusion, profuse sweating and
                            irritation of the bladder may occur with large
                            doses of methylene blue.

FURTHER READING

Gosselin RE et al. (1976) Clinical toxicology of commercial products, 4th edn. Williams and
    Wilkins, Baltimore
Harvey SC (1980) Methylene blue. In: Gilman AG, Goodman LS, Gilman A (eds) The pharmaco-
    logical basis of therapeutics, 6th edn. Macmillan, New York, p 980

1.23 Vitamins

When tonics are used for symptoms such as weakness and tiredness, stress,
"geriatric" conditions and "super potency", no physiological or pharmacological basis exists for such claims. Vitamins are appropriately used when
prescribed for the prevention or treatment of vitamin deficiencies.

Certain vitamin-mineral preparations contain as much as, or more than, 17%
alcohol. This amount of alcohol may be enough to encourage abusive
consumption by some persons. In patients using drugs such as disulfiram, an
acute acetaldehyde reaction may result.

Vitamin A (Retinol)

REQUIREMENTS   Vitamin A plays an essential role in the function
                           of the retina, and it is required for growth and
                           differentiation of epithelial tissue and bone, and
                           for reproduction and embryonic development.
                           The adult normal requirement of vitamin A is
                           supplied by an adequate diet. The rational use of
                           vitamin A is limited to the treatment of deficiencies
                           and to prophylaxis during periods of increased
                           requirements in infancy and early childhood, the
                           second and third trimesters of pregnancy, and
                           lactation (Table 1.15).

Table 1.15. Daily vitamin A requirements

Normal adult	Infants and growing children	Late pregnancy and lactation
Supplied by normal diet	400–700 retinol equivalents	1000–1200 retinol equivalents

Notes: 1. Supplements of vitamin A are not required for healthy adults.
2. 1 retinol equivalent = 1 μg of retinol = 3.3 units of vitamin A activity as supplied by β-carotene.
3. The maximum daily prophylactic dose of Vitamin A is of the order of 1200 retinol equivalents.

HYPERVITAMINOSIS A   Numerous freely available vitamin A preparations contain considerably higher amounts of vitamin A for daily intake than required. Repeated intake of vitamin A in excess may result in hypervitaminosis A (Table 1.16). Congenital abnormalities have been described in infants whose mothers have taken excessive amounts of vitamin A during pregnancy.

Vitamin A and its chemical analogues may be helpful in certain diseases of the skin such as acne, psoriasis and ichthyosis. Retinoic acid causes less liver toxicity than retinol.

Table 1.16. Features of hypervitaminosis A [based on Fisher KD et al. (1970) Dark adaptation and night vision. Fed Proc 29:1605]

Site	Clinical effects
General	Malaise, lethargy, tissue deposition of carotenoids
Skin and mucous membranes	Desquamation
Skeletal tissues and bone	Decalcification, fractures, early epiphyseal closure; hypercalcaemia; increased osteoblastic activity; cortical thickening and bone tenderness; raised serum alkaline phosphatase
Reproductive system	Resorption of embryos, congenital malformation
Nervous system	Increased intracranial pressure, which may result in the triad of headache, vomiting and papilloedema

Vitamin B$_{12}$ and Folic Acid

In view of the inter-relationship of these two vitamins, it is important that all preparations for therapeutic use that contain folic acid should also contain vitamin B$_{12}$. Increased intake of folic acid may mask vitamin B$_{12}$ deficiency, which may only become apparent when the more characteristic neurological lesions of the deficiency become manifest. Vegetarians and elderly subjects in whom vitamin B_{12} intake is very low are at particular risk. Large and repeated doses of folic acid may lower the blood concentration of vitamin B_{12}.

Increased folic acid intake in patients on long-term treatment with anticonvulsant drugs is thought to lead to destabilisation of epilepsy. This association is rare, and many epileptics have tolerated folic acid well.

It is unusual for folate and vitamin B_{12} deficiency to occur in isolation and they are more likely to be associated with multivitamin deficiencies. In such cases other vitamins and minerals (such as iron) may also need to be administered.

Vitamin C

ANTISCORBUTIC
ACTIVITY

Vitamin C (ascorbic acid) functions as a co-factor in certain essential biological reactions mainly involving oxidation and reduction. It is required for the synthesis of collagen and carnitine, and of steroids by the adrenal cortex, for the conversion of folic acid to folinic acid, and microsomal drug and tyrosine metabolism.

The therapeutic uses of vitamin C are in the prevention and treatment of scurvy (vitamin C deficiency). The normal daily antiscorbutic dose in adults and children over the age of 1 year is 50–150 mg. The higher dose is considered adequate to cover the majority of cigarette smokers who have higher vitamin C requirements than the normal population. For the treatment of a vitamin C deficiency disorder the dosage should be 500 mg. Higher doses than that are inadequately absorbed from the gastrointestinal tract.

There is no evidence that vitamin C prevents or ameliorates colds, or promotes wound healing. Likewise, claims for the therapeutic value of vitamin C in the following conditions, in the absence of vitamin C deficiency, are not supported by scientific data: atherosclerosis, allergy, mental disorders, schizophrenia, corneal ulcers, idiopathic methaemoglobinaemia, thrombosis, megaloblastic anaemia and capillary fragility.

TOXICITY

Consumption of vitamin C in excess of 1000 mg daily may be hazardous in some individuals. Oxalate, uric acid and calcium excretion in the urine may be increased, which in turn may cause crystal formation in the kidney, ureter or bladder. Patients with small intestinal disease, who may have increased urinary oxalate excretion, are at high risk of this potential complication.

Sodium comprises approximately 12% of the weight of sodium ascorbate. Patients in cardiac or renal failure may be at risk of developing hypernatraemia with excessive vitamin C intake.

Vitamin D

NORMAL REQUIREMENTS   The normal daily requirements of vitamin D are indicated in Table 1.17. Consumption above 2000 IU daily for prolonged periods may be associated with hypercalcaemia and nephrocalcinosis, and recurrent renal calculi have been noted in individuals ingesting no more than 1100 IU daily. Approximately 20% of normal adults who receive 100 000 IU of vitamin D daily will develop hypercalcaemia. The maximum safe dose of vitamin D has not yet been determined.

Table 1.17. Normal daily vitamin D requirements

Normal adult[1]	Growing children and pregnant women	Special populations[2]
100 IU	400 IU	400 IU

Notes: 1. Daily intake of vitamin D in adults in excess of 1000 to 2000 IU is likely to prove toxic in the long term.
2. This refers to elderly or cloistered individuals, food faddists, and persons of poor socioeconomic status for whom routine daily ingestion of vitamin D-containing foodstuffs is difficult.

INDIVIDUAL   A fairly wide range of individual susceptibility to
SUSCEPTIBILITY   the toxic effects of vitamin D exists. In growing children who may be taking calcium in amounts exceeding 1.0 g daily there may be a high degree of sensitivity, with hypercalcaemia and inhibition of growth developing on doses only 4–6 times greater than normal. In others the same effects may not develop after years of treatment.

In hypoparathyroidism and in patients with renal, chronic liver or biliary diseases the normal response to vitamin D may be diminished. Patients with sarcoidosis are prone to develop hypercalcaemia on very small doses of vitamin D.

HYPERVITAMINOSIS D   The effects of vitamin D toxicity are due either to acute hypercalcaemia and accompanying electrolyte abnormalities on cognitive functions, cardiac rhythm, renal and gastrointestinal function, or to indirect longer-term results of diffuse metastatic calcification in the kidney, heart and blood vessels. The symptoms associated with hypercalcaemia include weakness, fatigue, malaise, dry mouth, vague muscle and bone pain, headache and a metallic taste. Weight loss, diarrhoea, anorexia, nausea and vomiting reflect the gastrointestinal response to hypercalcaemia. Thirst, polyuria, nocturia, burning of the eyes, conjunctivitis, generalised pruritus, diminished libido, pancreatitis, renal calculi, photophobia, rhinorrhoea and hypertension may also develop. Hypertension, hemiplegia and mental impairment have been reported in children. It has been suggested that long-term consumption of vitamin D may be a predisposing factor in the development of myocardial infarction in man.

Vitamin K

Vitamin K promotes the hepatic biosynthesis of clotting factors II, VII, IX and X. The daily human requirement is extremely small, and needs are satisfied by the average diet and by synthesis of the vitamin in the intestinal tract.

ADVERSE EFFECTS   Side-effects of vitamin K are rare and have mainly been reported in the newborn with synthetic vitamin K_3, menadione, and its derivatives. Haemolytic anaemia, a raised serum bilirubin and kernicterus have been described, particularly in premature infants given large doses (5–30 mg daily).

TREATMENT OF   When vitamin K is used to correct hypoprothrom-
HYPOPROTHROMBINAEMIA   binaemia or bleeding secondary to anticoagulation the subsequent re-attainment of therapeutic levels of clotting factors may be difficult. The disorders for which the anticoagulants were being used, such as thrombosis or myocardial infarction, may deteriorate in the absence of adequate anticoagulation. For this reason the use of vitamin K is not recommended in anticoagulant-induced bleeding. The best approach to the management of the

excessive effects of oral anticoagulants is by titrated infusion of fresh frozen plasma.

In patients who have severe hepatic disease the damaged parenchymal cells may not be able to produce the necessary clotting factors, even if excess vitamin is available. For reasons which are not known, the administration of large doses of vitamin K or its analogues in an attempt to correct hypoprothrombinaemia associated with severe liver disease may result in a further depression of the concentration of prothrombin.

FURTHER READING

Labadarios D et al. (1978) Effects of chronic drug administration on hepatic enzyme induction and folate metabolism. Br J Clin Pharm 5:167

Federal Register, Food and Drug Administration (1979) Vitamin and mineral drug products for over-the-counter human use. 44:16, 126

2 Drug Safety in Some Common Medical Conditions

2.1 Heart Failure

The drug treatment of congestive cardiac failure is shown diagrammatically in Fig. 2.1. Most patients are effectively managed with diuretics and digitalis, and vasodilator agents have become an accepted second-line approach for patients who do not respond to standard therapy.

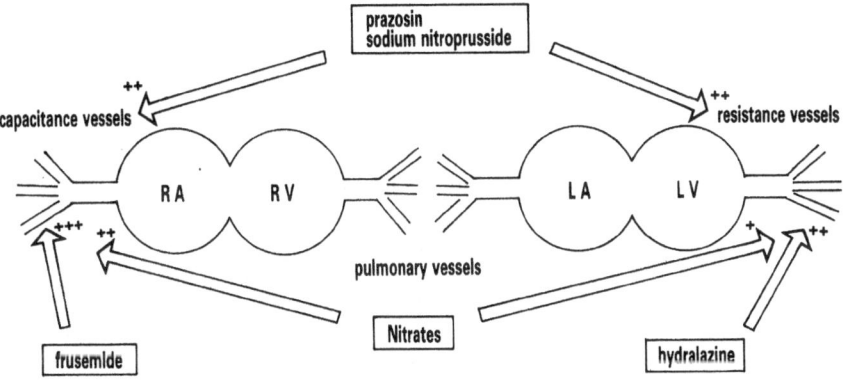

Fig. 2.1. Principles of drug management of congestive cardiac failure. *RA*, right atrium; *RV*, right ventricle; *LA*, left atrium; *LV*, left ventricle

The following are the main treatment-related problems experienced in the management of heart failure:

EXCESSIVE DIURESIS — Individuals differ widely in their response to diuretics, and an initial excessive diuresis may occur requiring the diuretic regimen to be tailored to the urinary output. After initial mobilisation of fluid with a potent, high-ceiling diuretic such as frusemide, treatment is normally continued with a thiazide or potassium-retaining diuretic.

The effects of excessive diuresis in this context are a falling urinary output associated with intravascular dehydration (which may occur despite peripheral oedema), a rising blood urea and serum creatinine, and a failure to maintain the initial response to treatment. Contraction alkalosis may result (Fig. 2.2).

DIURETIC ESCAPE

"Diuretic escape" may develop with long-term therapy, manifesting itself as a diminished response. As the main diuresis in congestive cardiac failure is characteristically at night (due to redistribution of fluid in the supine position) diuretic therapy may have to be administered at night, despite the inconvenience that this may cause. Judicious salt restriction may be useful in refractory patients. When splanchnic venous congestion is severe, the bioavailability of thiazides and loop diuretics may be reduced. Parenteral rather than oral administration of a diuretic over a short period may circumvent the problem.

HYPOKALAEMIA

Depletion of total body potassium is the most common complication of intensive diuretic therapy. Besides the debility that may result, cardiac function may be reduced and dysrhythmias precipitated. When digitalis is taken concomitantly with diuretics, hypokalaemia may "sensitise" the diseased heart to the toxic effects of digitalis, resulting in severe arrhythmias, conduction disturbances, or combinations of these, even when serum levels of digitalis are within normal limits.

DIGITALIS TOXICITY

This is discussed on p. 30. Digitalis toxicity may aggravate congestive cardiac failure.

MYOCARDIAL
ISCHAEMIA

An excessive fall in arterial pressure induced by vasodilators (uncommon in severe failure) may jeopardise myocardial perfusion. The effects of vasodilators on coronary resistance, particularly in diseased vessels, are unpredictable. A steal effect may be created from diseased vessels which may be maximally dilated to non-diseased vessels

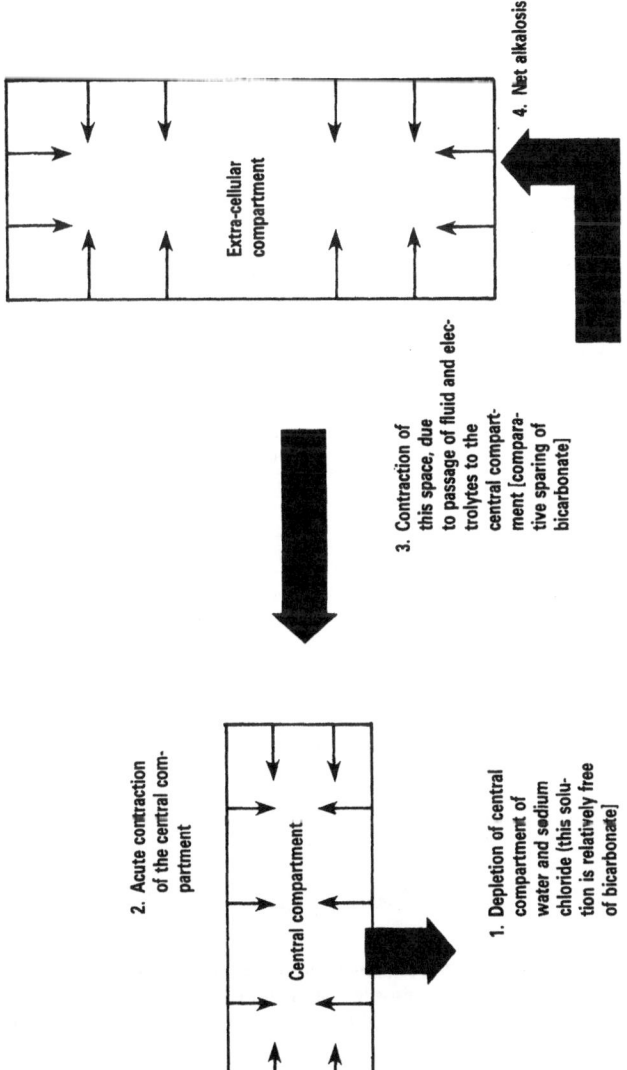

Fig. 2.2. The pathogenesis of diuretic-induced contraction alkalosis.

which can still respond to dilation. Evidence as to whether vasodilators exacerbate or improve function and metabolism of ischaemic myocardium is conflicting.

ADVERSE DRUG–DRUG
INTERACTIONS

Several drug combinations may depress myocardial contraction or impair atrioventricular conduction in patients with heart failure (see Table 2.1).

Table 2.1. Adverse drug-drug interactions in heart failure

Interacting drugs	Possible consequences
Digitalis / diuretics	Diuretic-induced hypokalaemia predisposes to digitalis cardiotoxicity
Digitalis / β-blockers	Combined depression of atrioventricular conduction, with danger of heart block
Digitalis / quinidine or disopyramide	Depression of atrioventricular conduction. Quinidine may raise serum digoxin levels
Digitalis / verapamil	Sinoatrial and atrioventricular block may be produced, particularly with intravenous verapamil.

Note: See also Fig. 2.3.

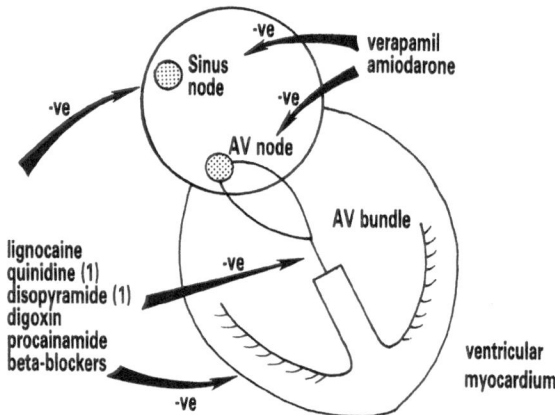

Fig. 2.3. Potential adverse, drug-drug interactions in the treatment of disorders of the heart. [1] These anticholinergic agents may, in toxic doses, also cause acceleration of atrioventricular conduction.

LACK OF RESPONSE TO
THERAPY

In patients with congestive cardiac failure not responding *ab initio* to therapy, or whose initial response is not maintained despite continued treatment the following possible reasons should be considered:

i) Drug therapy may be insufficient (dosage, lack of compliance).

ii) Drug therapy may be inappropriate (digitalis toxicity, diuretic escape, drug-drug interaction, inadvertent use of a negative inotropic agent such as a β-blocker).

iii) Electrolyte abnormalities (hypokalaemia, hyponatraemia and hypomagnesaemia may all render cardiac failure refractory to therapy).

iv) Persistence of aggravating factors (pulmonary emboli; pulmonary, urinary tract or other infections; anaemia; arrhythmias).

v) Failure to remove the cause (hyperthyroidism, progressive ischaemia, progressive rheumatic carditis, cardiomyopathy, viral myocarditis).

vi) Development of complications (deep vein thrombosis, with or without pulmonary emboli; sepsis; bacterial endocarditis).

No patient can be regarded as suffering from refractory cardiac failure until these possibilities (particularly those that are treatable) have been rigorously excluded.

FURTHER READING

Mason DT (1978) Vasodilator and inotropic therapy of heart failure. Am J Med 65:101
Opie LH (1980) Drugs and the heart. Lancet, London

2.2 Hypertension

Antihypertensive drug therapy should be undertaken with due regard to the following *general considerations*:

1. The aim of treatment is to restore the blood pressure to normotensive levels if possible. (The elderly hypertensive is an exception; see p. 144).

2. With most antihypertensive agents, including the diuretics, the dose-response curve alters at doses higher than the maximum recommended; thus they are unlikely to influence the blood pressure further, and the safety-benefit ratio may be altered disadvantageously.

3. There is evidence that the incidence of the following complications of hypertension is reduced by appropriate antihypertensive therapy:

i) Stroke, especially cerebral haemorrhage

    ii) Subarachnoid haemorrhage
   iii) Congestive heart failure
    iv) Malignant hypertension
     v) Renal failure
    vi) Dissecting aortic aneurysm
   vii) Progression to a more severe stage

4. There is no clear evidence that the incidence of the atherosclerotic complications of hypertension is altered by control of the disease.

STEPPED APPROACH TO   Figure 2.4 shows diagrammatically the stepped
DRUG TREATMENT   approach to the drug treatment of hypertension,
                           with the details expanded in the notes which
                           follow.

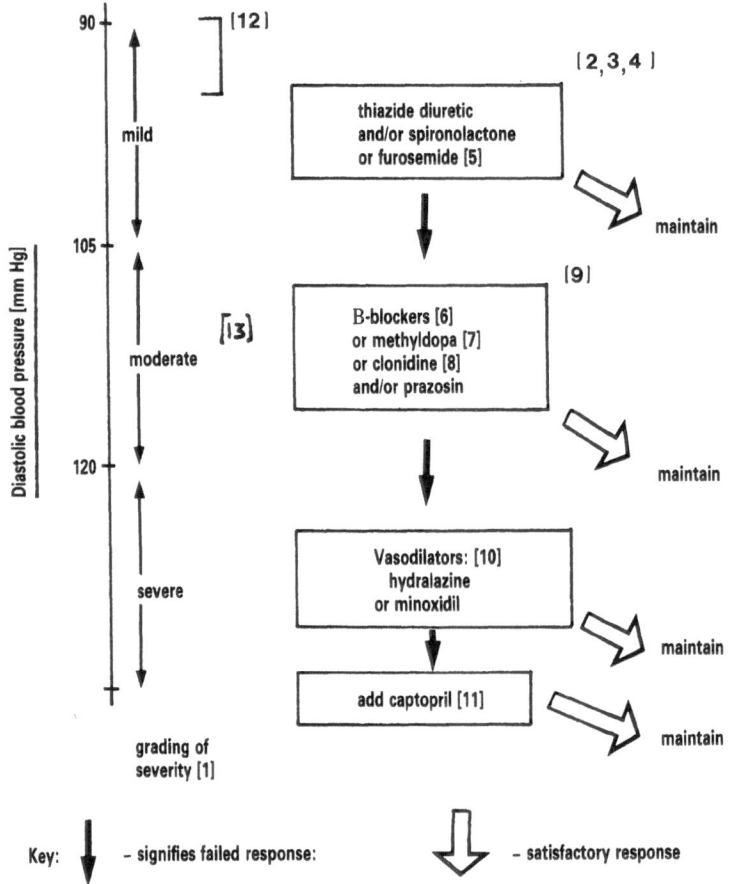

Fig. 2.4. Stepped approach to the treatment of hypertension (Numbers refer to the following notes.)

Notes:

1. The grading of severity of hypertension is according to the Joint American Committee (1977) JAMA 237:255.

2. Diuretics are used first in this approach as they are often effective alone in mild and moderate hypertension, they may be given in a daily dose, they are inexpensive, and side-effects are usually not serious.

3. The effective daily antihypertensive dose range of the diuretics concerned is of the following order:

Thiazides:

chlorothiazide	500–1000 mg
hydrochlorothiazide	25– 100 mg
chlorthalidone	25– 100 mg
Spironolactone	50– 400 mg
Frusemide	20– 100 mg

4. Thiazide diuretics, if they are going to be effective, are likely to lower the blood pressure within 3–4 days. The beneficial effects may be due to alteration of sodium balance or direct arteriolar dilatation, or both. Spironolactone, the aldosterone antagonist, is as effective as thiazides when given in high doses and is a useful alternative when thiazides are contraindicated.

5. Frusemide causes greater fluid and electrolyte disturbance than the thiazides and it is usually reserved for patients with associated heart failure when other diuretics are not effective.

6. The prototype β-adrenergic blocking drug is propranolol. It blocks all β-receptors: cardiac (β_1), arteriolar (β_2) and bronchiolar (β_2). Cardioselective β-blockers such as metoprolol and atenolol have less effect on bronchial and peripheral vascular smooth muscle and may be of value in moderate doses in patients with asthma, heart failure or peripheral vascular disease. In higher doses the β_2-receptor agonists lose their selectivity. Long-acting β-blockers such as nadolol or atenolol, which have a prolonged half-life, have the advantage of being effective in once-daily dosage.

7. Methyldopa, a false neurotransmitter, decreases sympathetic vasomotor outflow from the central nervous system. Individual responses vary and the drug is effective in lowering blood pressure only 50% of the time.

8. Clonidine is similar to methyldopa in mechanism of action except that it is not a false neurotransmitter.

9. Recommended dosage ranges for second-step antihypertensive agents are of the order indicated below:

Propranolol	40– 480 mg
Timolol	20– 60 mg
Nadolol	40– 320 mg
Metoprolol	50– 400 mg
Methyldopa	500–2000 mg
Clonidine	0.1– 2 mg
Prazosin	1– 20 mg

There is little point in exceeding the maximum daily recommended antihypertensive doses as further benefit is unlikely to accrue and the disadvantages may become correspondingly more prominent.

10. Hydralazine is not used alone because its direct relaxing effect on vascular smooth muscle, which lowers peripheral resistance, also increases renin secretion, with resultant retention of salt and water and expansion of plasma volume. Hydralazine is effectively combined with a diuretic and a β-blocker.

    For a discussion of minoxidil see p. 83.

11. For a discussion of captopril see p. 80.

12. *Mild hypertensives.* The evidence is insufficient to permit a clear statement to be made as to which of these patients should be treated, and by what drugs. It is not certain that treatment

reduces mortality in this group, although it appears likely that this is the case. (Little is known about the natural history of mild untreated hypertension.) Not all mild hypertensives require treatment. However, the following factors are associated with a higher risk of morbidity and mortality and should probably indicate selection for treatment:

Younger age group	—	younger patients are at greater risk than the older age group.
Race	—	in the United States of America the mortality due to hypertension is higher in blacks than in whites.
A family history of hypertension		
Lability	—	the prognosis in patients with labile blood pressure and large fluctuations is likely to be better than when a raised blood pressure is less labile.

13. All patients with a diastolic pressure exceeding 105 mm Hg should be treated.

CAPTOPRIL

Captopril is the first of a new class of antihypertensive drugs with a competitive inhibitor action on angiotensin converting enzyme which converts angiotensin 1 to angiotensin 2. Despite this specific mechanism of action captopril has been effective in patients with hypertension regardless of whether renin levels are high, low or normal. It may be effective alone, but because of its toxicity it is reserved for patients who have failed to respond satisfactorily to multidrug regimens, or who have developed unacceptable side-effects from other agents. A thiazide-type diuretic will be necessary in addition in most patients. The blood pressure lowering effects of captopril and thiazides appear to be additive. Captopril and β-blockers seem to have a less than additive effect.

Within the first few hours of the initial dose of captopril patients on diuretic therapy may occasionally experience a precipitous reduction in blood pressure. This is most likely when intravascular volume has been depleted by diuretic therapy, severe dietary salt restriction or haemodialysis. An initial transient hypotensive response is not a contraindication to further treatment.

Captopril shares certain chemical similarities with penicillamine, and the toxicity profile of the drug is similar. Neutropenia, proteinuria and a self-limiting skin rash are the most common side effects. A membranous glomerulopathy has been identified, and a described association of this with a serum sickness-like syndrome suggests immune complex deposition as a basis for the pathology.

The occasional neutropenia induced by captopril has been associated with myeloid hypoplasia.

Characteristically this is cumulative after numerous weeks of therapy, and is likely to reverse on discontinuation of the drug. Often there has been associated systemic lupus erythematosus or another autoimmune collagen disorder. It is advised that particular caution should be exercised if the white blood count should fall below 4000/ mm^3 or if the white blood cell count falls to 50% of the pre-treatment level in a patient receiving captopril.

Proteinuria in excess of 1 g per day has been noted in a small proportion (approximately 1%) of patients treated with captopril. The nephrotic syndrome has occurred in a minority of such patients. Most cases of proteinuria have occurred within the first 9 months of treatment, suggesting the importance of surveillance in this regard in the early stages of treatment. Increasing proteinuria calls for re-evaluation of the treatment. In most cases proteinuria can be expected to subside after discontinuing the drug.

METHYLDOPA

Treatment with α-methyldopa is associated with a high incidence of side-effects, which are usually mild but may occasionally be severe. The most frequent are manifestations of central nervous system depression. Drowsiness and changes in mental activity with a decrease in concentration may result in mistakes in professional activities and an impaired capacity to drive a motor vehicle. There have been reports of amnesia-like episodes. Such effects may occur in patients taking normal doses, and they may not be readily detectable unless patients are questioned carefully. They are especially likely in renal failure, when elimination of the drug may be impaired.

Inappropriate acute hypotensive responses to methyldopa are common in patients with renal impairment and in the elderly. Rarely hypotension may be incapacitating.

Methyldopa hepatotoxicity is well documented. A picture resembling hepatitis with acute onset is commonest; there is hepatocellular damage and sometimes cholestasis. Massive liver cell necrosis with a fatal outcome after re-exposure following previous liver toxicity has been described. The hepatitis normally resolves after discontinuation of the drug, but a disease resembling chronic active hepatitis can ensue. α-Methyldopa is contraindicated in patients with a history of liver disease.

Fever associated with symptoms resembling an infectious illness has been described in about 3% of patients treated. The fever characteristically develops in the first few weeks of treatment. It is not clear whether continued administration under such circumstances predisposes the patient to other complications, but this has to be assumed (see section on drug fever, p. 155).

Several unique immunological abnormalities may complicate long-term therapy with α-methyldopa: the appearance of a Coombs-positive immunoglobulin, and occasionally haemolytic anaemia; antinuclear and rheumatoid factors may appear in the serum; and elevations of immunoglobulin A, immunoglobulin G and immunoglobulin M levels may be noted.

Impairment of sexual function in men, with decrease in libido and failure of ejaculation, is common.

BETA-ADRENORECEPTOR BLOCKING AGENTS

See p. 39.

FRUSEMIDE

The efficacy of frusemide as an antihypertensive agent is controversial. There is no convincing evidence that frusemide is superior to thiazides in the treatment of hypertension, with the possible exception of hypertension associated with chronic renal failure and severe fluid retention. Hypertension which is not controllable with a thiazide diuretic alone is unlikely to respond to frusemide.

PRAZOSIN

The haemodynamic effects of this α-adrenergic blocking agent in patients with hypertension and congestive cardiac failure are due to its action as a peripheral vasodilator. (The drug has a similar molecular structure to both cyclic adenosine 3′,5′-monophosphate and the direct smooth muscle relaxing agent papaverine.)

Postural hypotension after the first dose administration is related to dose and to intravascular volume depletion (see p. 38). Other side-effects seldom limit therapy. Due in part to its selective α-adrenergic receptor antagonism (see Fig. 1.9) the hypotensive effect of prazosin is accompanied by little or no increase in heart rate, plasma renin activity, or plasma noradrenaline concentration. This is a distinct advantage over non-selective α-adrenergic antagonists.

MINOXIDIL

Minoxidil causes vasodilation by a direct effect on vascular smooth muscle. It is potent and potentially toxic, and has proved valuable in the treatment of patients with severe symptomatic or organ-damaging hypertension that cannot be managed with other agents. It has a valuable place in the treatment of patients with severe hypertension and end-stage renal disease, when the only alternative management would be bilateral nephrectomy. In a small number of patients with malignant hypertension, marked and sustained improvement in renal function has been achieved with minoxidil. It is generally accepted that minoxidil should never be used for primary treatment.

The fluid and sodium retention caused by minoxidil may be difficult to control even with large doses of a potent diuretic. The mechanism of this effect is not certain. Generalised oedema and even brain swelling may result, necessitating withdrawal of the drug. If given alone the potent vasodilator effect of minoxidil may activate the adrenergic nervous system. Tachycardia and angina pectoris may be precipitated. For this reason minoxidil is usually given with β-blockers to control tachycardia.

Approximately 80% of patients receiving minoxidil develop hirsutism, and in women particularly this may be to an extent that is unacceptable.

DRUG TREATMENT IN THE ELDERLY

Reference is made on p. 144 to the principles of treatment of hypertension in the elderly subject.

Diuretics are usually well tolerated. The potassium-conserving diuretics can cause a dangerous hyperkalaemia, particularly if they are given together with potassium supplementation.

β-Adrenergic blocking drugs can cause fatigue and lassitude, which may lead to a state of clinical or subclinical depression. There may be a reduction in exercise capacity, and peripheral vasoconstriction as a result of β-blockade may adversely affect an already compromised peripheral circulation. It may be that β-blockers which have limited access to the central nervous system (such as atenolol or nadolol) may cause less central nervous system depressive effects than other more lipid-soluble agents. Despite these drawbacks the β-blockers can be valuable in the elderly hypertensive patient.

α-Adrenergic blocking drugs tend to cause severe postural hypotension in older patients who already have reduced plasma volumes and impaired baroreceptors, and in whom there is a danger that posture-related hypotension may significantly reduce cerebral perfusion.

FURTHER READING

Adler S (1974) Methyldopa-induced decrease in mental activity. JAMA 230:1428
Colucci WS (1982) Prazosin review. Ann Intern Med 97:67
Editorial (1975) Side effects of methyldopa. Br Med J I:646
Editorial (1980) Minoxidil. Med Lett Drugs Ther 22:21
Editorial (1980) Captopril. Lancet II:129
Food and Drug Administration Drug Bulletin (1981) Captopril. 11:10
Hoorntje SJ et al. (1980) Immune complex glomerulopathy with captopril. Lancet I:1212
Linas SL Niles AS (1981) Minoxidil. Ann Intern Med. 94:61
Medical Letter on Drugs and Therapeutics (1972) Drugs in hypertension. 14:63
Mitchell HC et al. (1980) Renal function during long-term treatment of hypertension with minoxidil. Ann Intern Med 93:676

2.3 Cough

Cough is useful for clearance of the respiratory tract of foreign material and excess secretion; not uncommonly, however, it may be non-productive and irritating. When sputum is produced it may be undesirable for a cough to be suppressed, but when a dry nocturnal cough interferes with sleep, such as may happen in terminal carcinoma of the lung, it should be controlled. Treatment of the cough of acute bronchitis and pneumonia is seldom necessary if appropriate antibiotic therapy is initiated in time; suppression of cough in chronic bronchitis and bronchiectasis is undesirable except when it is non-productive and interferes with sleep.

Theoretically, a cough may be blocked peripherally, at sensory receptors in the respiratory tract, at the afferent arc, centrally in the nervous system at the cough centre, and at the efferent arc. In practice, *cough suppressants* are regarded as either peripheral-acting or central-acting, and often their precise action is not known. Morphine, codeine and other opiate alkaloids are thought to raise the threshold of the cough centre to tussive stimuli; of the peripheral-acting agents some have local anaesthetic actions, others a bronchodilator effect (bronchospasm is thought to be a contributory factor to cough), and others mucokinetic and hydrating actions. The action of placebos is little understood.

Morphine is the prototype of the cough suppressants, although codeine is preferred for its wider therapeutic margin. Certain non-narcotics also have a central antitussive action. There is a danger with opiates that they may induce sputum retention and reduce mucokinesis, and thus in patients with impaired central respiratory drive ventilatory failure may result. The opiates are regarded as dangerous in bronchial asthma. (This is universally accepted in the case of morphine, but the position regarding less potent cough sedatives in asthma merits further definition.) All are likely to cause severe constipation, and because of dependence potential the opiates are excluded from chronic use except in patients with incurable disease. The opiates are metabolised in the liver, and patients with impaired liver function may be at particular risk of toxicity. (This may also be explicable in terms of undue receptor sensitivity.) The effects of the narcotic antitussives are summarised in Table 2.2.

Table 2.2. Narcotic antitussives (based on Ziment 1978)

Drug	Antitussive effect	Analgesic effect	Sedative effect	Respiratory depression	Addiction potential	Adult dose (mg)	Duration of effect (h)
Heroin (diacetylmorphine)	++	++	++	++	++		3–4
Morphine	++	++	++	++	++	2–4	4–5
Codeine (methylmorphine)	++	+	±	+	±	5–20	4–6
Hydrocodone (dihydrocodeinone)	++	+(?)	+	+	++	5–10	4–8
Oxycodone (dihydrohydroxy-codeinone)	++	+	+	+	++	3–5	4–5
Methadone	+	++	++	+	+	2.5–10	3–5
Morpholinylethyl-morphine (pholcodine)	+	±	±	+	−	5–15	4–5
Meperidine (pethidine)	±	++	+	+	+	25–50	2–4

CODEINE   Codeine is the methyl ester of morphine; it has weak analgesic activity and is considered less toxic than morphine in humans, although it is more so in many animals.

Equal antitussive doses have approximately 1/20 the psychic effect of morphine; thus, codeine presents a comparatively small risk of dependence. It may be that the abuse potential of codeine is greater when it is used in conjunction with central nervous system sedatives or stimulants. As a pro-drug which converts in the body to morphine, codeine may depress the respiratory centre in the elderly and other sensitive subjects. Even low doses may cause constipation, nausea, vomiting, drowsiness, and occasionally paradoxical excitement and agitation. High doses have the toxic effects of morphine.

There is no scientific basis for the use of *expectorant cough mixtures,* and no agent is known which has a selective action on the cough reflex to facilitate expectoration. If these agents have an effect at all, it is probably a result of placebo action. The combined use of cough suppressant and expectorant seems illogical.

MUCOLYTIC AGENTS

Bromhexine, acetylcysteine and sodium mercapto-ethane sulphonate (mesna) are used to liquify the sputum. Their efficacy is not convincing. Bronchorrhoea and/or bronchospasm may occasionally result from a local irritative or allergic effect, but these compounds are generally well tolerated in asthmatics.

ANTIHISTAMINES

Several studies have demonstrated the antitussive efficacy of antihistamines, usually in doses that cause appreciable drowsiness. A potential risk of respiratory centre depression exists.

FURTHER READING

British National Formulary (1981) No 2. British Medical Association and The Pharmaceutical Society of Great Britain, London, p 94
Hughes DT (1978) Cough suppressants. Br Med J I:1202
Irwin RS et al. (1977) Review of cough. Arch Intern Med 137:1186
Ziment I (1978) Respiratory pharmacology and therapeutics. Saunders, Philadelphia

2.4 Bronchial Asthma

METHYLXANTHINES

Aminophylline and theophylline are widely used in the treatment of bronchial asthma, and also in chronic obstructive airways disease. Their efficacy and safety are dose-dependent and subject to considerable inter-individual variations, being affected by age, body weight and pathological conditions such as pulmonary and heart diseases, and even apparently by acute asthma itself. Absorption from the gastrointestinal tract of aminophylline preparations is highly variable between subjects, but control has been improved by sustained-release oral preparations and by continuous intravenous infusion and blood level monitoring in critically ill patients. In patients with hepatic cirrhosis and with acute pulmonary oedema the rate of elimination of theophylline has been shown to be prolonged more than six-fold compared with healthy adults (in whom the $t_{1/2}$ of elimination is of the order of 8–9 h). This prolongation probably reflects the renal clearance of the drug in a situation in which there is no appreciable hepatic metabolism. It follows that patients with reduced hepatic function or hepatic perfusion should receive lower doses, and in subjects at risk it is recommended that the blood level should be determined regularly if treatment is continued beyond 10–12 h. On the other hand, a major problem with the use of methylxanthines can be suboptimal administration with a corresponding lack of effect.

The methylxanthines are active cerebral cortical stimulants (although aminophylline is least potent of the group in this regard) with additional stimulatory actions on the medullary respiratory centre, the circulatory system, and the smooth muscles of the bronchi. Both the therapeutic and adverse responses derive from these pharmacological effects.

Excessive dosage or undue sensitivity to aminophylline and theophylline result in nervousness, nausea, vomiting, dizziness and convulsions. Insomnia, restlessness and excitement are early symptoms which may progress to delirium. Sensory disturbances such as ringing in the ears and flashes of light may be experienced. The muscles become tense and tremulous. Focal and generalised seizures can occur without prior signs of toxicity. Seizures are usually associated with very high plasma levels, such as a theophylline level exceeding 40 μg/ml, although convulsions and death have resulted at concentrations as low as 25 μg/ml. In many respects the cerebral effects of methylxanthines are similar to those of the sympathomimetic agents (see p. 33).

An association can usually be found between tachycardia and toxic plasma concentrations of theophylline. Tachycardia is a reliable indicator of toxicity, as opposed to nausea and vomiting, which do not necessarily bear a relationship with high plasma levels. A risk of ventricular tachycardia and fibrillation, as well as supraventricular arrhythmias, exists in these circumstances. Extrasystoles are common when plasma concentrations of theophylline are high. The appreciable reduction in theophylline elimination in patients with compromised cardiac function puts these patients at risk of serious toxicity. In the worst case hypertension or hypotension may result, and any disturbance in blood pressure may aggravate the cardiac status causing cardiac output to fall, leading to eventual cardiac and vasomotor collapse. A hazard of rapid intravenous administration of aminophylline is sudden death, which is probably of cardiac origin. It may be that precipitation of free theophylline at the pH of the blood results in high local concentrations which are responsible for cardiac toxicity. Slow injection over at least 20 min helps to avoid this.

Although oral preparations of aminophylline and theophylline cause irritation in the gastrointestinal tract, manifesting as nausea and vomiting, these symptoms are as much a function of the plasma concentration, and they are not obviated entirely by parenteral administration. Taken with food oral preparations may cause less local irritation in the gastrointestinal tract; at the same time their absorption is likely to be slow, although not reduced. Patients with active peptic ulceration tend to tolerate the methylxanthines poorly.

Based on these considerations several guidelines

for the effective and safe use of aminophylline and theophylline suggest themselves:

i) In patients with acute bronchospasm a loading dose is generally required and this is most safely administered intravenously over not less than 20 min.

ii) Particular care is required in young children, old people, in patients with hepatic impairment, in the presence of cardiovascular disease including cor pulmonale, or where there is central nervous system excitation, because such patients may be especially sensitive to the toxic effects of these medicines.

iii) The drugs have to be given cautiously and in reduced dosage if theophylline-containing agents have been taken in recent days.

iv) If it is necessary to prescribe intravenous therapy for several days, changes in the dosage regimen are based on the clinical response and appearance of side-effects such as nausea, vomiting, tachycardia or central nervous system irritability, and it may be necessary to modify dosage according to the progress of the acute illness.

v) It is difficult to achieve optimum results in maintenance therapy using a fixed dosage regimen. Periodic review and adjustment of the prescribed dose is often necessary. In a particular individual considerable variation can be expected.

vi) There is no accepted pharmacological basis upon which one theophylline or aminophylline preparation can be recommended rather than another. Although there is some evidence to suggest that long-acting preparations provide superior control of bronchospasm compared with the short-acting agents, their main advantage is one of convenience of dosing.

vii) There is seldom a necessity for chronic administration by any route other than the oral, although occasional patients seem to have a better clinical response with rectal administration.

COMBINATION
ANTI-
ASTHMATIC
PREPARATIONS

The addition of ephedrine to aminophylline or theophylline is widely considered undesirable, as it is likely to increase the side-effects without making any marked contribution to the bronchodilator effect.

Although it is common practice to add barbiturates to a methylxanthine preparation there are many disadvantages, including the possibility of inducing enzymes that may bring about more rapid degradation of the active drugs used to treat bronchospasm.

Expectorant drugs are incorporated in many products, although these are usually present in subtherapeutic amounts. Furthermore, they are likely to increase gastric irritation and nausea.

The evidence for greater than additive therapeutic responses to combinations of β_2-adrenergic agonists and theophylline or aminophylline is not convincing, although individualised regimens of combinations of these two classes of agents may well achieve effective bronchodilation with less risk of toxicity than is currently the general experience. There remains some controversy in this area.

In general it can be said that the use of preparations with fixed-dose combinations of components is not rational unless they chance to correspond to an optimised regimen previously established for the individual patient with the agents concerned. Such preparations limit the physician's manoeuvrability in achieving for the patient the ideal dosage of theophylline or its congeners or derivatives, using empirical guidelines and clinical judgement.

FURTHER READING

Editorial (1979) Theophylline in asthma. Drug Ther Bull 17:91
Jacobs ME et al. (1976) Theophylline kinetics. JAMA 235: 1983
Rall TW (1980) Theophylline. In: Gilman AG, Goodman LS, Gilman A (eds) The pharmacological basis of therapeutics, 6th ed. Macmillan, New York, p. 592
Ziment I (1978) Respiratory pharmacology and therapeutics. Saunders, Philadelphia

2.5 Tuberculosis and Other Mycobacterial Infections

In the treatment of tuberculosis and other mycobacterial infections there is an initial intensive phase in which at least three bactericidal drugs are administered in order to achieve cure. Ideally, intensive therapy should be continued for at least 8 weeks and until the sensitivities of the organism have been established. This minimises the chance of development of resistant strains.

Subsequent therapy is continued with two or three drugs, selected if possible on grounds of the sensitivity of the organism, for a total duration of 9 months. Regular review is essential.

DRUGS OF CHOICE   First- and second-line drugs are indicated in Table 2.3.

Table 2.3. Drugs in the treatment of mycobacterial infections

Mycobacterium	Drug order of choice	
	1st	2nd
M. tuberculosis	Rifampicin[1] Streptomycin Isoniazid (INH)[3] Ethambutol Pyrazinamide[4]	Ethionamide[2] Cycloserine[2]
Mycobacteria other than M. tuberculosis[5]	Ethionamide[2] Cycloserine[2] Rifampicin Ethambutol[6]	Isoniazid Streptomycin
M. lepra	Dapsone Rifampicin	Clofazimine

Notes: 1. Rifampicin is normally given to patients with miliary and organ (non-pulmonary) tuberculosis, including tuberculous meningitis, and to high-risk subjects.
2. These agents are comparatively less bacteriostatic and more toxic than the first-line antituberculous drugs.
3. 10–20% of M. tuberculosis are INH-resistant in certain parts of the world.
4. The special indications for pyrazinamide are re-treatment of pulmonary tuberculosis and short-course chemotherapy.
5. These mycobacteria are variably sensitive to the standard first-line agents.
6. These mycobacteria are variably sensitive to ethambutol.

TREATMENT FAILURE   Treatment failure may be primary or secondary. Alcoholics, diabetics, patients undergoing treatment with corticosteroids, individuals who have had a previous partial gastrectomy, associated chronic debilitating disease, and those with large residual cavities in the lungs are all at special risk of developing tuberculosis and not responding to therapy.

Other important causes of failure are:

i) Irregular drug ingestion (compliance in the treatment of tuberculosis is all important);

ii) Primarily resistant *Mycobacterium tuberculosis* organisms (very unusual); and

iii) Atypical mycobacteria (e.g. *M. fortuitum* and *M. kansasii*), which are often resistant to standard drugs.

Sensitivity testing of the organism is of particular importance in these cases. Relapses generally occur within 6 months of stopping treatment and are managed in the same way as a newly diagnosed patient. First-line drugs should be re-used if the bacillus is sensitive to them, and rifampicin should be added if it has not already been used. If ethambutol is prescribed in re-treatment higher doses are given than those used initially (e.g. 25 mg/kg per day for 2 months, followed by 15 mg/kg per day).

TOXICITY PROFILES

The toxicity profiles of the commonly used antituberculous drugs are given in Table 2.4.

RENAL FAILURE

An important problem in the treatment of tuberculosis is the dosage adjustment which is necessary in patients with impaired renal function. In Table 2.5 guidelines are set out for adjustment of dosage schedule according to the degree of renal decompensation.

HEPATOTOXICITY

Drug injury to the liver is a common complication of antituberculous therapy. Isoniazid, rifampicin, pyrazinamide, and, less commonly, ethambutol are potentially hepatotoxic. A degree of cross-sensitivity exists between ethionamide, isoniazid and pyrazinamide. Liver injury usually occurs in the first 3 months of therapy, indicating the importance of close surveillance for this complication during the early months of therapy.

Premonitory symptoms and signs (indicating the allergic nature of this drug reaction) are fever, skin rash, lymphadenopathy, arthralgia, eosinophilia and atypical monocytosis in the peripheral blood. The clinical picture may be confused with viral hepatitis.

Diagnosis is made on clinical grounds, and an elevation of serum glutamic oxaloacetic transaminase (SGOT) to three times normal, or the association of a raised SGOT, serum bilirubin and/or

Table 2.4. Toxicity profiles of the antituberculous drugs

Antibiotic	Adverse effects	Comments
Isoniazid (INH)	i) Acute viral hepatitis-like reaction; the aetiology of this is not clear ii) Hepatitis, dose- and age-related; characteristically occurs in patients over 35 years of age. An increased risk is identified in alcoholics; underlying liver disease and concurrent rifampicin therapy may have fatal outcome iii) Neurotoxicity; polyneuritis, mental disturbance, confusion, psychosis, convulsions (rare)	The relationships between slow acetylator status and peripheral neuropathy, and fast acetylator status and hepatotoxicity have been disputed
Ethambutol	Retrobulbar neuritis (rare with the recommended dosage; related to dose and accumulation in the body) Special risk factors: poor renal function poor eyesight young age pregnancy	Dosage reduction is necessary in renal failure. Monthly examination of visual acuity and red-green colour discrimination is required
Pyrazinamide	Hepatotoxicity is the most important adverse effect. This is unlikely to develop with moderate dosage and short-term (weeks) therapy. It is dose-related and a higher incidence is associated with long-term therapy. Clinically the picture resembles that caused by INH	
Rifampicin	i) Hepatotoxicity is common (up to 20% of cases). Patients with underlying liver disease, and those receiving concomitant therapy with other hepatotoxic drugs are at particular risk ii) An unexplained flu-like syndrome may be seen, particularly when rifampicin has been given long term or intermittently in high dosage. iii) Allergic cutaneous syndromes	The dose of rifampicin should be reduced in hepatobiliary disease. Mild elevation of hepatic enzymes in the serum may be noted early in the course of treatment. This does not necessarily reflect hepatotoxicity, and they may return to normal with continued therapy

Table 2.5. Dosage adjustments of antituberculous drugs in renal decompensation

Drug	Major excretion route	t½ (h) normal	t½ (h) ESRD	Normal dose interval (h)	Adjustment of dosage interval for renal failure Creatinine clearance		
					>50	10–50	<10
Streptomycin	Renal	2.5	100–110	12	24(h)	24–72(h)	72–96(h)
Isoniazid	Hepatic (renal excretion of metabolites)	2–4 (slow acetylators) 0.5–1.5 (rapid acetylators)	4	24	Unchanged	Unchanged	66–100(h)
Rifampicin	Hepatic	2–5	2–5	24	Unchanged	Unchanged	Unchanged
Ethambutol	Renal	4	8	24	24(h)	24–36(h)	48(h)
Ethionamide	Knowledge incomplete; only 1% excreted in urine as active drug	2–4	2–4	8	Unchanged	Unchanged	Unchanged
Pyrazinamide	Primary renal	?9–10	?	8	?	?	?

ESRD = end stage renal disease

alkaline phosphatase. The SGOT should be monitored regularly in the early months of antituberculous treatment. Liver biopsy is of little value in distinguishing a drug effect from viral hepatitis. The mortality from hepatic failure or severe haemorrhage is high, and it is very important that treatment is discontinued immediately warning signs appear.

There is good evidence that combined therapy with isoniazid and rifampicin may cause a particularly severe form of hepatotoxicity, with a worse prognosis than that attributable to either drug alone.

It frequently happens that hepatotoxicity develops in patients who are in need of continued therapy. Corticosteroids are of little value in this situation, and they may be harmful, both from the point of view of the hepatic injury and the tuberculosis. In such an event therapy should be discontinued and the drugs reintroduced serially, starting with that which is considered least likely to be responsible for the hepatotoxicity. The commencing dose in each case should be approximately one-tenth the normal daily dose. Progressive daily increments are given until the appropriate dosage is reached, with careful monitoring of clinical state and hepatic enzymes. After a week's therapy on full dosage the next drug in line is reintroduced in a similar manner.

PREGNANCY

When the pregnant mother develops tuberculosis, treatment should not be withheld because of concern regarding a teratogenic effect of therapy. Experience shows that the first-line drugs, isoniazid, ethambutol and rifampicin have a reasonable margin of safety when used during pregnancy. Over 90% of pregnant women treated for tuberculosis with these drugs can expect to deliver normal infants. Amongst the antituberculous drugs streptomycin is associated with the highest incidence of malformations in the developing fetus. Approximately one in six newborns exposed in utero to streptomycin can be expected to have some hearing loss or vestibular defect. The risk of this effect of streptomycin exists throughout gestation.

A widely accepted approach to the treatment of tuberculosis during pregnancy appears to be that, if the disease is not extensive, isoniazid is used in combination with ethambutol and pyrazinamide. Streptomycin is given by most authorities in the first phase of the treatment. If a more potent drug is necessary, because of the extensive or serious nature of the disease, rifampicin may be added.

FURTHER READING

Girling DJ (1982) Adverse effects of antituberculous drugs. Drugs 23:56
Joint Tuberculosis Committee of the British Thoracic and Tuberculosis Association (1973) Chemoprophylaxis of tuberculosis. Tubercle 54:309
Kucers A, Bennett NMcK (1979) The use of antibiotics, 3rd edn. Heinemann, London
Rossouw JE, Saunders SJ (1975) Hepatotoxicity. Q J Med 44:1
Snider DE et al. (1980) Treatment of tuberculosis during pregnancy. Am Rev Respir Dis 122:65

2.6 Fungal Infections

AMPHOTERICIN B

This is a polyene antibiotic to which *Cryptococcus neoformans, Candida albicans* and *Aspergillus* are usually sensitive. *Actinomyces* and *Nocardia* species are not sensitive. Development of resistance to amphotericin B is not a common problem in practice. Systemic fungal infections are treated intravenously.

Amphotericin B is toxic. During infusion, fever, chills, headache, anorexia, nausea, vomiting and sometimes hyperthermia may be marked. Local thrombophlebitis is common. Certain of these effects can be obviated if small doses of heparin and hydrocortisone are added to the infusion, and oral or intramuscular antihistamine or chlorpromazine may be of value.

Nephrotoxicity is the most important adverse effect of parenteral amphotericin B. The drug causes some impairment of renal function in almost all cases. This is manifested by a rise in blood urea and serum creatinine, and a fall in creatinine clearance, associated with the appearance of red and white blood cells, albumin and casts in the urine. Nephrotoxicity frequently limits the duration of treatment with amphotericin B, but the drug can usually be continued without undue danger until blood urea levels rise higher than 7.1 mmol/l. Early renal damage related to amphotericin B is reversible. Permanent impairment of renal function appears to be related to the total dose used, and it is estimated that this is likely in 40% of patients who receive a cumulative total of more than 4 g. The possibility of amphotericin nephrotoxicity should not preclude its use in patients with potentially fatal systemic fungal infections, if this is the only suitable drug available.

The mechanism of the nephrotoxicity and strategies for its prevention are not well understood.

Hypokalaemia due to excessive renal tubular loss of potassium is a common and early feature of amphotericin B toxicity. Potassium supplements are required for most patients receiving the drug.

A normochromic normocytic anaemia associated with reduced erythropoiesis may complicate therapy with amphotericin B. This is usually reversible on cessation of the drug, but there are occasions when the anaemia is severe enough to require treatment by blood transfusion. Thrombocytopenia has occasionally been noted, but leucopenia is very rare.

Intrathecal and intraventricular administration may be indicated in patients with cryptococcal meningitis not responding to intravenous therapy. Severe arachnoiditis can follow. The drug is a potent neurotoxin and besides chemical meningitis it may cause peripheral nerve pain, paraesthesiae, nerve palsies, paraplegia and convulsions. Intraventricular administration is thought to be less likely to result in chemical meningitis than intrathecal therapy.

5-FLUOROCYTOSINE

5-Fluorocytosine is related structurally to 5-fluorouracil. There is evidence that the combination of 5-fluorocytosine and amphotericin B results in supra-additive activity against *Cryptococcus neoformans* and against sensitive strains of *Candida*. The development of resistance in a large proportion of patients restricts the use of the drug as single treatment. The mechanisms of this resistance are not understood. Its action in fungal cells appears to be based on its conversion to fluorouracil by an enzyme; this fluorinated pyrimidine has cytotoxic activity.

Metabolism of 5-fluorocytosine to 5-fluorouracil may account for the leucopenia and thrombocytopenia which are sometimes noted with the drug. It is rapidly and well absorbed from the gastrointestinal tract and excreted largely unchanged in the urine. The dosage should be altered in patients with renal insufficiency (see Table 2.6). An underlying malignancy or haematological disorder, or concurrent or prior therapy with radiation and/or cytotoxic drugs, predispose to the bone marrow depressant effect of this agent.

In severe systemic fungal infections 5-fluorocytosine is commonly used together with amphotericin B.

Table 2.6. Dose adjustment of antifungal drugs in renal failure [reproduced with permission from Bennett WM et al. (1980) Drug therapy in renal failure. Ann Intern Med 93:62]

Antifungal drug	Pharmacokinetic variables								
	Major excretion route	Half-life ($t_{1/2}$)		Normal dose interval (h)	Volume of distribution (l/kg)	Adjustment for RF[a] cl.creat.			Removed by dialysis
		Normal (h)	ESRD (h)			>50	10–50	<10	
Amphotericin B	Non-renal	24	24	24	4	24	24	24	No
5-Fluorocytosine	Renal	3–6	70	6	0.6	6	12–24	24–48	Yes
Miconazole	Hepatic (renal)[b]	20–24	20–24	8	?	Unchanged			No

Key: ESRD = end stage renal disease; RF = renal failure; cl.creat. = creatinine clearance
[a]Refers to interval adjustment of dose (in hours) in renal failure
[b]Lesser pathway of elimination

FURTHER READING

Diasio RB (1978) 5-Fluorocytosine. Antimicrob Agents Chemother 14:903
Sande MA (1980) Antimicrobial agents. In: Gilman AG, Goodman LS, Gilman A (eds) The pharmacological basis of therapeutics, 6th edn. Macmillan, New York, p 1233
Kucers A, Bennett NMck (1979) The use of antibiotics, 3rd edn. Heinemann, London

2.7 Malaria

Drug considerations in the treatment of malaria are indicated in Fig. 2.5.

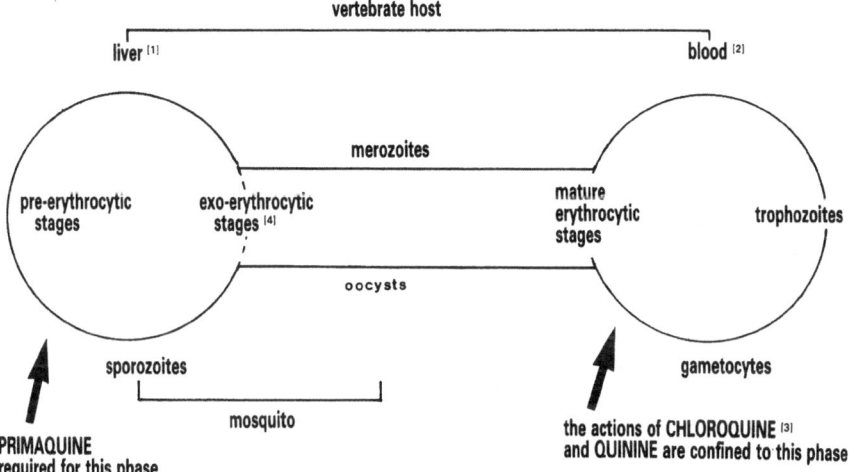

Fig. 2.5. Schematic representation of the plasmodial life cycle and principles of management. (Numbers refer to the following notes.) [Reproduced with kind permission from Rollo IM (1964) The chemotherapy of malaria. In: Hutner SH (ed) Biochemistry and physiology of protozoa, vol III. Academic Press, New York, p 525]

Notes:

1. Chloroquine does not eliminate the liver stage in malaria due to *Plasmodium malariae*, *P.vivax* and *P.ovale*. Additional treatment with primaquine (15 mg/d for 14 days) is necessary to achieve eradication of the hepatic phase of the disease. It is given either with or after the completion of the chloroquine course.

2. *P. falciparum* is confined to this phase. The parasite does not enter an hepatic cycle. Primaquine may be given in *P.falciparum* infestations to cover the possibility of concurrent infection with other plasmodia.

3. In Southeast Asia and Central and South America, and to a limited extent in East Africa, *P.falciparum* may be resistant to chloroquine. Treatment is with quinine or mefloquine.

4. Refers to relapsing malarias only.

CEREBRAL MALARIA

This is associated with a heavy infestation of *Plasmodium falciparum*. Cerebral malaria does not exist in isolation—renal, liver and cardiac failure are invariably associated.

Treatment of cerebral malaria (and of any severe infestation of *P.falciparum*) is with quinine or chloroquine given intravenously in glucose-saline infusions.[1] Quinine and chloroquine given together may be antagonistic.

There is no good evidence in support of the use of

---

[1]Quinine 0.65 g in 500 ml glucose-saline given intravenously over 2–4 h, three times daily until the patient can take drugs orally; or 150 mg chloroquine intravenously in glucose-saline, as for quinine.

corticosteroids or intravenous dextran in cerebral malaria, and heparin may be harmful by extending the effects of the consumptive coagulopathy and bleeding that are associated.

ADVERSE EFFECTS OF ANTIMALARIAL AGENTS

Occasionally quinine infusion may cause neurological toxicity such as twitching of the lips, shaking, delirium, confusion and even convulsions and coma.

Such effects may be difficult to distinguish from those of cerebral malaria, and they may aggravate the clinical picture. Intravenous chloroquine may have similar neurotoxic effects.

Primaquine given in large doses to individuals with red blood cell glucose-6-phosphate dehydrogenase (G6PD) deficiency may precipitate acute haemolysis. (G6PD-deficient patients can usually tolerate eight weekly doses of 45 mg of primaquine.)

PROPHYLAXIS IN PREGNANCY

All agents used in malaria prophylaxis are known to cross the placenta.

If possible, a woman should not enter a known malaria region during the first trimester so that the question of prophylaxis need not arise. If a woman lives in a malaria zone or if a visit to one is unavoidable, then one of the following drugs can be considered:

Chloroquine. No congenital malformations appear to have been reported with the low dose required for malaria prophylaxis (500 mg once weekly). However, in patients receiving higher doses throughout pregnancy cochlear damage has been reported in the offspring.

Pyrimethamine interferes selectively with folate metabolism in the parasite and might cause repercussions in the fetus, for whom folic acid metabolism is important. It is considered safe in a prophylactic dose of 25 mg per week. Should the pregnant woman's folate status be compromised, folinic acid (citrovorum factor, Calcium Leucovorin, United Kingdom) may be used concurrently. Folinic acid bypasses the pyrimethamine blockade of folate metabolism. Folic acid will not protect in these circumstances.

Dapsone is not recommended in pregnancy, especially as it is only available in combination with pyrimethamine, which presents a double attack on fetal folate metabolism.

Quinine is a well-known teratogen and is not advised.

FURTHER READING

Bruce-Chwatt LJ (1974) Transfusion malaria. Bull WHO 50:337
Hall AP (1976) Quinine-chloroquine interaction. Br Med J I:323

2.8 Urinary Tract Infections

With modern antibiotics eradication of the invading micro-organism in urinary tract infections (UTI) is relatively simple to achieve when the urinary tract is structurally normal; in contrast, it is difficult to eliminate the same organism in the presence of a calculus or when infection is localised to the prostate gland. The infecting organism is likely to be an *Escherichia coli. Klebsiella pneumoniae, Proteus mirabilis* and other *Proteus* species, *Streptococcus faecalis* and *Enterobacter aerogenes* are other organisms commonly identified with UTI:

Several general statements can be made which have relevance to the drug therapy of uncomplicated UTI:

1. Microbiological and sensitivity testing are of value in planning therapy, and quantitative urine cultures may be necessary to differentiate the urethral syndrome from bacterial cystitis or pyelonephritis.

2. Relief of clinical symptoms does not necessarily indicate cure, which can only be ascertained by confirming elimination of bacteriuria after therapy has been completed.

3. Community-acquired infections, and particularly first infections, are likely to be caused by antibiotic-sensitive organisms.

4. Uncomplicated infections confined to the lower urinary tract (urethra, bladder) are likely to respond to low doses and short courses of antimicrobial therapy, whereas upper urinary tract infections require longer periods of treatment. (The difficulty in practice is location of the infection. Antibody coating of bacteria is likely to help, but this laboratory test is not generally available.) For infections involving the kidneys, which are associated with systemic symptoms, antibiotics which provide effective blood and tissue levels are required (see Table 2.7).

Table 2.7. Concentration of oral antibacterial agents in the urine and blood (Bailey 1974)

Agent	Adequate concentrations	
	Urine	Blood
Sulphonamides	Yes	Yes
Cotrimoxazole	Yes	Yes
Ampicillin	Yes	Yes
Amoxicillin	Yes	Yes
Nitrofurantoin	Yes	No
Nalidixic acid	Yes	No
Methenamine	Yes	No

ANTIMICROBIAL
THERAPY OF
UNCOMPLICATED
INFECTIONS

Cotrimoxazole, ampicillin, nitrofurantoin, nalidixic acid or a sulphonamide appear to be comparably effective in uncomplicated UTI. Trimethoprim and cotrimoxazole (trimethoprim with sulphamethoxazole) have produced similar cure rates in several reported studies. For a first episode a 7-day course of treatment is likely to be sufficient. Single dose therapy with ampicillin or cotrimoxazole has proved successful in treating cystitis.

Table 2.8. Causes of relapsing urinary tract infections

Cause	Comment
1. Wrong choice of drug	If the antibiotic sensitivity of the organism is not known, the best guess in general practice would be ampicillin or cotrimoxazole (depending upon prevalent faecal organisms of the population concerned)
2. Emergence of resistant strains	This may occur during treatment if inadequate drug concentrations are achieved. This is most likely in the presence of impaired renal function
3. L-forms	Antibiotics which act by interference with bacterial cell wall synthesis (e.g. penicillins, cephalosporins) may produce L-forms. These can survive in the hypertonic conditions of the renal medulla. Once treatment is stopped L-forms may revert to their bacterial form. Suggested management of persistent L-form infection is with agents which are active against cell wall-defective organisms (e.g. erythromycin)
4. Urolithiasis	Micro-organisms can be cultured from the centre of calculi removed from patients with UTI; these organisms are likely to be protected from antibacterial agents. Long-term treatment may be necessary if symptomatic relapses continue after removal of stones
5. Prostatic infection	Many commonly used antibacterial agents fail to penetrate prostatic fluid, or may not be effective in the acidic prostatic fluid. Erythromycin, oleandomycin, cotrimoxazole, tetracycline and clindamycin achieve concentrations in the prostate high enough to achieve therapeutic effect

REPEATED INFECTIONS

Repeated infections may be either relapses or reinfections. The former are caused by the same microorganism and they usually occur within a month of cessation of therapy. A relapse may be due to inappropriate drug selection, inadequate dosage, emergence of resistance or patient failure to take the prescribed treatment.

When recurrent infection is due to relapse, and if irremedial abnormalities of the renal tract are present, long-term therapy is widely advocated. Surgical correction of structural abnormalities may be necessary.

The important causes of relapsing UTI are indicated in Table 2.8.

As a rule a relapse is due to an upper tract focus. Anatomical abnormalities and urolithiasis have to be excluded in patients who fail to respond to standard therapy.

Reinfection is a new infection caused by a different organism. Repeat short-term therapy is appropriate for patients who are reinfected.

CATHETER-ASSOCIATED INFECTIONS

Optimum treatment regimens for catheter-associated UTI have not been established. These often remit spontaneously or with short-term antibiotic therapy if the catheter can be removed. If that is not possible, systemic antibiotics or urinary antiseptics may reduce bacteriuria, but are unlikely to eliminate it.

Asymptomatic bacteriuria in catheterised patients is generally regarded as unlikely to progress to serious infection. Therefore vigorous drug therapy is not warranted in patients who are not immunosuppressed or who are not at high risk of sepsis because of structural abnormality of the urinary tract, diabetes mellitus, or other disease.

TREATMENT IN RENAL FAILURE

Infections in patients with acute or chronic renal failure are commonly hospital-acquired and likely to be caused by resistant organisms. Therapeutic concentrations of antibacterial agents in the urinary tract may be difficult to attain without systemic toxicity due to impaired renal handling of the drug concerned. Disparity of function of the kidneys may lead to unequal excretion of antibacterial agents with persistence of infection in the kidney with the poorer function.

NALIDIXIC ACID

Nalidixic acid is bactericidal to most of the common Gram-negative bacteria that cause UTI. It is less effective against Gram-positive micro-organisms, and *Pseudomonas* species are resistant to its action. Acquired resistance develops readily during therapy, but does not appear to be transferable. It has been estimated that 25% of patients with UTI harbour micro-organisms primarily resistant to nalidixic acid.

High concentrations of nalidixic acid and its active metabolite, hydroxynalidixic acid, are achieved in the urine but not in the prostate gland. Whether nalidixic acid effectively penetrates the renal medulla and is of value in the treatment of pyelonephritis is uncertain.

Nalidixic acid has been used successfully in the treatment of acute UTI. The follow-up cure rate in patients with chronic infections is disappointing. With prolonged therapy, resistant bacterial strains emerge in a high proportion of cases.

Oral nalidixic acid is usually well tolerated, but nausea, vomiting and abdominal pain may occur. Neurotoxic reactions such as headaches, vertigo, visual disturbances, and even convulsions (which may be on the basis of intracranial hypertension) have emerged when this drug has been used in large doses. It seems wise to use it cautiously in patients in renal failure (when the normal half-life of 8 h may be prolonged to 21 h), and in patients with pre-existing mental instability, epilepsy and cerebral arteriosclerosis.

NITROFURANTOIN

Nitrofurantoin mainly acts within the lumen of the urinary tract. Due to reabsorption in the distal tubules the renal tissue level is higher than that achieved in other tissues.

This drug is a furan, and furans in general may be toxic to liver cells. Necrosis may result. Acute hepatocellular injury and cholestatic jaundice have been described in association with the drug. Chronic active hepatitis in women, with positive antinuclear antibodies in the majority of cases, has been described on numerous occasions. The situation is similar to that produced by α-methyl-dopa. The majority of patients have improved clinically after withdrawal of the drug; cirrhosis has developed in a small number.

Nitrofurantoin induces pathological lung reactions more commonly than all other drugs combined. Women are mainly affected, particularly those in middle age. An acute allergic reaction, independent of dose, may follow sensitisation 1–2 weeks earlier. Within a matter of hours after re-intake an acute illness may develop which is characterised by a high fever, skin rash, non-productive cough, severe dyspnoea, tachypnoea, chest pain, frequently cyanosis, and not uncommonly collapse. There may be acute shock.

Chronic interstitial pulmonary reactions to nitrofurantoin are 10–20 times less common than acute ones. During long-term medication a clinical picture of increasing dyspnoea and cough, usually unproductive, without fever or acute symptoms may evolve. The clinical findings are dense râles usually heard over the basal regions, and commonly a restrictive respiratory impairment and interstitial infiltrations on X-ray. Symptoms can be expected to regress promptly upon nitrofurantoin withdrawal. In most cases the radiological findings recede more slowly and resolution is incomplete in almost half the patients. Rarely, because of marked fibrosis, resolution does not occur at all. There is little evidence that corticosteroids are of value in the treatment of patients with the chronic pulmonary form of nitrofurantoin toxicity.

As opposed to the acute nitrofurantoin lung reaction, which probably constitutes an immune complex type of allergic response, the aetiological basis for the chronic reaction is not understood at all.

Nitrofurantoin is neurotoxic, and cases of severe peripheral neuropathy have been described directly attributable to it. Pathological evidence of severe axonal degeneration has been found. The polyneuropathy characteristically starts peripherally, predominantly affecting the limbs. It remains more severe distally. Initially there is sensory loss with paraesthesiae; later motor loss develops, often with severe muscle atrophy. In advanced cases the process is not reversible and the patient may remain an invalid. The pathogenesis of this injury is unclear. Degenerative changes include anterior horn cells and muscle fibres as well as myelinated nerves. Although the neuropathy is not necessarily dose-related and not clearly linked with degree of abnormality of renal function, it is generally accepted that renal impairment is a contraindication to use of the drug because of an association with its neurotoxic potential.

FURTHER READING

Bailey RR (1974) Review of UTI. Drugs 8:54
Gleckman R et al. (1979) Nalidixic acid. Am J Hosp Pharm 36:1071
Holmberg L et al. (1980) Adverse reactions to nitrofurantoin. Am J Med 69:733
Jayasundera NS et al. (1980) Chronic pulmonary reaction to nitrofurantoin. JAMA 243:769
Sussman M, Asscher AW (1970) Urinary tract infection. In: Black D, Jones NF (eds) Renal
    disease, 4th edn. Alden, Oxford, p 400
Yiannikas C et al. (1981) Nitrofurantoin neuropathy. Aust NZ J Med 11:400

2.9 Cancer Chemotherapy

The antineoplastic agents have amongst the lowest therapeutic indices of any drugs, and as such they cause frequent and predictable multi-system toxicity. The adverse effects are acute, such as extravasation, emesis, mucositis, alopecia, and depression of the bone marrow; or delayed and dose-related, such as pulmonary disease, cardiotoxicity, infertility and malignant change.

Many antineoplastic drugs, particularly the alkylating agents, are irritant to the skin and subcutaneous tissues if they *extravasate* inadvertently. Intense local inflammation and necrosis may result. A small risk of extravasation exists even when chemotherapy infusions are administered by trained staff.

Virtually every chemotherapeutic agent causes *nausea and vomiting*. Usually the discomfort is mild, but emesis may be severe, and can persist for up to 48–72 h. This frequently becomes the major dose-limiting feature of a drug regimen. Fluid and electrolyte disturbances, and chronic anorexia and nutritional impairment may result from periodic nausea and vomiting; less commonly violent retching results in Mallory-Weiss oesophageal tears or collapse of metastatically involved vertebrae.

Acute cytotoxic damage to the lining of the *gastrointestinal tract* is, with bone marrow suppression, the most severe toxic expression of antineoplastic agents. Oral mucositis is most common, perhaps because of the rapid cell proliferation of the oral mucosa and its vulnerability to direct trauma. Susceptibility to oral mucositis may also be related to oral hygiene, but this association has not been confirmed. Oesophagitis, diffuse ileitis and colitis may occur. Diminished fluid and food intake, and occasionally malabsorption may result.

The effect on cell proliferation is likely to reduce renewal of mucosal cells, resulting in atrophy and ulceration. Such reactions are dose-related, although there is considerable patient variation. Stomatitis and ulceration may also result from drug-induced neutropenia; when mucositis and neutropenia occur in association the local defence to micro-organisms is altered, and there is danger of local as well as disseminated infection.

Many chemotherapeutic agents regularly cause *alopecia* in a dose-related manner. The majority of hair follicles are in growth phase, so that after multiple courses of cytotoxic therapy virtually all follicles will be affected. Affected hair fibres contain fewer cells per unit length and they become thin and fragile, breaking off soon after emerging from the follicle. The injury to the follicle is temporary, and normal hair growth will resume following cessation of therapy. A period of 2–4 months may be required for regrowth. Occasionally hair follicles become resistant to chemotherapy and patients may grow hair through subsequent treatment cycles.

A wide variety of *acute allergic reactions*, ranging from brief febrile episodes to hypersensitivity reactions, which include erythematous rashes, vesicular or bullous eruptions, erythema multiforme and exfoliative dermatitis, have been associated with various antineoplastic agents. Fortunately such reactions are uncommon, with the exception of L-asparaginase, which is an immunogenic enzyme of bacterial origin.

The use of the anthracycline antibiotics in cancer chemotherapy has been linked with the development of *cardiomyopathy*, and recent reports suggest that numerous anticancer agents may have cardiotoxic effects in humans. Doxorubicin (Adriamycin, United Kingdom) is the anthracycline antibiotic which has been most consistently associated with this complication. It is relatively rare, dose-related, and of late onset (that is, after months of therapy). Other antitumour drugs and regimens which have been linked with cardiotoxicity include actinomycin D, and radiation when this is directed to the mediastinum. Combined treatment with potentially cardiotoxic agents may produce additive or synergistic effects.

Long-term administration of corticosteroids and prolonged use of busulfan for chronic myeloid leukaemia have been associated with development of *posterior subcapsular cataracts*. The pathogenesis and the reason for the localisation are not clear; it may be that drug damage to proliferating lens epithelial cells manifests posteriorly in the lens due to the normal migration of these cells in that direction. The cell damage may be caused by decreased DNA synthesis or perhaps, in addition, a drug-related interference with delivery of nutrients through the anterior lens epithelium to the remainder of the lens. The clinical and pathological changes in cytotoxic-induced cataracts are similar to cataracts associated with long-term steroid therapy for other conditions, and old age.

The course of steroid-induced cataracts after discontinuing therapy is variable. There may be regression; on the other hand, progression has been reported. Cataract surgery may be necessary if interference with vision is advanced.

Cytotoxic drugs are a major cause of *depression of the bone marrow*, resulting in leucopenia, agranulocytosis, thrombocytopenia and anaemia. Clinical symptoms and signs vary with the severity and rate of development of neutropenia, thrombocytopenia and anaemia. Haemorrhagic and infective manifestations are prominent in acute cases. The time relationship between exposure to therapy and onset of symptoms varies, and is generally dose-related. Bone marrow histology may be aplastic, but more often it is hypoplastic and there may be patches of normal or increased cellularity. (A single bone marrow biopsy may therefore be misleading.)

Thrombocytopenia may develop as part of an aplastic anaemia, or alone. The latter may result either from marrow depression or increased peripheral destruction. Many cytotoxic drugs which cause aplastic anaemia are also associated with thrombocytopenia. Bleeding is unlikely to occur spontaneously with a platelet count above 40 000/mm^3; between 10 000 and 20 000/mm^3 spontaneous bleeding is common, and below 10 000/mm^3 it is usual and often severe. In most cases bleeding takes place in the skin and mucous membranes. Bleeding into internal organs is uncommon, but is likely to be hazardous, particularly in the brain. Headache may be the first warning sign, and death may result from intracerebral haemorrhage. The true mortality of severe thrombocytopenia is estimated at less than 5 per cent.

Cessation of therapy does not necessarily result in rapid improvement of the blood count. There appear to be two patterns of bone marrow recovery following the administration of cytotoxic agents—rapid and delayed. Nitrogen mustard, cyclophosphamide, methotrexate, cytosine arabinoside and vinblastine tend to be associated with rapid recovery, whilst with carmustine and melphalan there is more often a delayed response.

As far as is known, cytotoxic drugs do not have long-term adverse effects on *fertility* in women. In men they may cause a profound reduction in sperm count. This tends to happen uniformly after treatment. Follow-up studies indicate that recovery usually occurs, although it may be delayed for several years. Infertility cannot simply be attributed to treatment itself, since it may also be related to a pre-existing deficiency in spermatogenesis or sperm transport. The alkylating agents chlorambucil, melphalan, cyclophosphamide, nitrogen mustard and busulfan have definitely been linked with a depressant effect on spermatogenesis, and procarbazine, cytosine arabinoside and vinblastine are regarded as probably having a similar effect.

Many cytotoxic drugs are mutagenic, and they carry a potential risk of producing *malignant change*. In ovarian carcinoma the incidence of acute non-lymphatic leukaemia after treatment has been reported to be increased 20-fold; in Hodgkin's disease a second malignancy is about 14 times more likely than the expected incidence. However, these must be seen in context of the therapeutic advantages gained by the treatment concerned.

Pulmonary toxicity caused by antineoplastic drugs is becoming a more frequently recognised entity, and the number of drugs known or suspected of causing this complication is increasing. It may be caused by cytotoxic drugs used singly or in combination. Direct toxicity probably accounts for most cases, but the mechanism(s) is uncertain. In some cases immune complexes may deposit in lung tissue causing tissue destruction. Drug damage to the heart or blood vessels and pulmonary embolism may contribute to the pathology.

The initial clinical appearance of chemotherapy-related pulmonary toxicity includes fever, dyspnoea and a non-productive cough with pulmonary râles. There may be X-ray evidence of alveolar or interstitial disease, or both, and occasionally of a pleural reaction. Weakness and weight loss occur in the majority of patients. Pulmonary function studies in advanced cases are likely to demonstrate hypoxaemia, restrictive ventilatory defect, and decreased diffusion capacity. A biopsy is usually necessary to confirm the diagnosis. Once symptoms and roentgenological signs have developed, the prognosis is likely to be poor, and the condition irreversible.

RESISTANCE TO
CYTOTOXIC AGENTS

Resistance may be primary (a non-responsive tumour) or acquired. The latter may resemble antibiotic resistance of bacteria.

GENERAL GUIDELINES

i) Given the present limited understanding of the pathophysiology of the nausea and vomiting effects of chemotherapy, and the restricted therapeutic armamentarium available for its control, careful pre-treatment patient preparation and treatment of complications by trial and error with available antiemetic medications remain the cornerstones of current therapy (see the section on antiemetic therapy, p. 173). Correction of fluid and electrolyte balance is essential in patients who are vomiting or not taking sufficient fluids.

ii) The risks of drug extravasation are reduced if patients report immediately any stinging or burning pain during infusion, or swelling or erythema at infusion sites. Infusions should be administered in anatomical regions with extensive soft tissue in order to avoid involvement of underlying tendons, nerves and blood vessels in the event of extravasation.

Care has to be taken that potentially necrotising drugs are administered through a freshly inserted intravenous line with a demonstrable blood return. For similar reasons, topical application of cytotoxic agents to the eye, nares, or other mucous membranes, or to the skin close to these structures, can be dangerous.

iii) The cardiomyopathy associated with doxorubicin is related to the cumulative dose received. In patients treated with a total dose of less than 550 mg/m² the risk of congestive cardiac failure is small (approximately 1%), but this increases sharply (up to 25%) at higher cumulative doses. It has been advised that patients who have received prior radiation therapy to the mediastinopericardial area should not be given more than 400–500 mg/m² of doxorubicin. The incidence of cardiomyopathy may be lower in patients given doxorubicin by infusion over a period of 30 min than when it is given rapidly. There is a danger that concern regarding this association may lead to under-utilisation of this important cytotoxic drug.

iv) The use of scalp tourniquets or local cooling to reduce blood flow has been proposed during chemotherapy to prevent alopecia. Although delay or reduction in alopecia has been reported for certain drugs, a theoretic objection exists that such techniques may render the scalp a "protected sanctuary" for future recurrent disease, and for this reason these approaches have been prohibited in many centres.

v) Prophylactic measures to prevent mucositis have been unsuccessful. Mouthwashes and intensive oral hygiene have been of limited use in control of secondary infection. It is important that nutrition and hydration are carefully protected. Treatment of stomatitis once it has developed is palliative with topical anaesthetics and mouthwashes.

vi) It is unwise to attempt conception when one partner is being treated with cytotoxic agents. It is not known what the "safe period" is after cessation of therapy, but 4–6 months has been proposed.

vii) For most tumours combination chemotherapy is more effective than single-agent therapy. Such combinations include drugs which are active when used alone against the specific tumour type. If they have different mechanisms of action increased cell kill may be achieved. If side-effects are different these should not be additive, and the combination is not likely to be more toxic than if the drugs are given singly. Figure 2.6 gives an indication of the chief site of action of the various cytotoxic drugs.

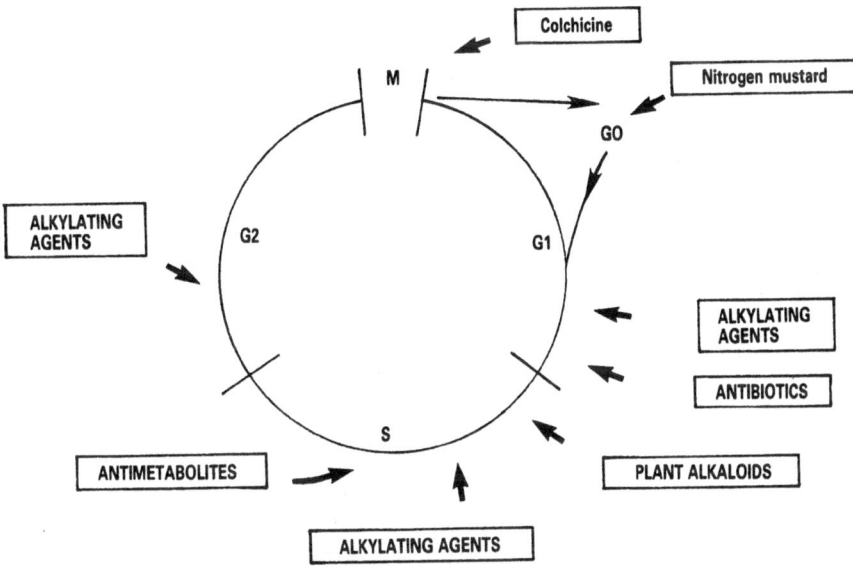

Fig. 2.6. The cell cycle and phase specificity of some cytotoxic drugs. M, mitosis; GO, resting phase of cell cycle; cells are not in cycle but capable of proliferation; S, phase of DNA synthesis and chromosome replication; G1, pre-replicative phase, involving operations preliminary to S-phase. RNA and protein synthesis continue normally; no DNA synthesis. Burst of RNA synthesis in late G1; G2, post-replicative, pre-mitotic phase. Relatively short and fairly fixed in duration.

Note: This is a simplification of the main actions of the antimitotic agents, and represents only their chief site of action. The distinction between these categories of actions of drugs, although fairly clear-cut in animal experiments, is oversimplified and presently of limited importance in human cancer. Most attempts at clinical kinetic scheduling have been unsuccessful. A common procedure is to employ non-cycle specific drugs followed by phase-specific agents, since the former may reduce the non-proliferating cell pool, which stimulates the survivors to enter mitosis when they can be killed by the phase-specific drug.

FURTHER READING

Batist G, Andrews JL (1981) Pulmonary toxicity of antineoplastic drugs. JAMA 246:1449
Griffin JD, Garnick MB (1981) Eye toxicity. Cancer 48:1539
Praga C et al. (1980) Cardiac toxicity from antitumour therapy. Oncology 37 Suppl 1:51

Rogers HJ et al. (1981) Cancer chemotherapy. In: A textbook of clinical pharmacology. Hodder and Stoughton, London, p 714
Spiegel RJ (1981) Acute toxicities of chemotherapy. Cancer Treat Rev 8:197
Thachil JV et al. (1981) Cancer and cancer therapy on fertility. J Urol 126:141

2.10 Iron-Deficiency Anaemia

When iron is given orally in the treatment of iron-deficiency anaemia it approaches the ideal form of medication—cheap, highly effective, with a clearly measurable response and a low order of toxicity. Medication alone will not suffice unless the underlying pathology responsible for the disturbance in iron balance has been identified and treated. With all forms of iron therapy given in appropriate doses in iron-deficiency anaemia a daily response in haemoglobin in excess of 0.1 g/dl can be expected from the fourth day of treatment, i.e. more than 2 g/dl over a 3-week period. (A haemoglobin response of 0.2 g/dl per day reflects red blood cell synthesis three times the normal rate.)

CONTRAINDICATIONS TO IRON

Unless there is clear indication of a deficiency of iron the administration is contraindicated in the following conditions: haemolytic anaemias, hypoplastic anaemia, sideroblastic anaemia, thalassaemia, chronic inflammation, and the anaemia of chronic renal disease. There is a risk of iron overload and the development of siderosis if such patients receive iron unnecessarily.

FAILED RESPONSE

In a patient with iron-deficiency anaemia who fails to respond satisfactorily to adequate doses of medicinal iron only a limited number of possible explanations exists: lack of compliance; mixed anaemia due to a combination of vitamin B_{12} and/or folic acid deficiency with iron depletion; coexistent infection; continued blood loss of the order of 20 ml or more daily; or failed absorption of iron from the gut (this is rare, and usually associated with steatorrhoea).

It is inappropriate to switch to more expensive or to parenteral forms of iron before these possibilities have been ruled out.

CHOICE OF AN ORAL IRON PREPARATION

The commonly used preparations such as ferrous fumarate, gluconate, succinate and sulphate differ only marginally in the degree of absorption of iron. Ferric salts are less well absorbed from the gut. Haemoglobin regeneration rate is little affected by the particular salt used, and for most patients there is no urgency to correct the haematological status. The choice of preparation can usually be decided on considerations of cost and the side-effects which may be experienced idiosyncratically.

There is no evidence that additives such as vitamin C significantly improve the intestinal absorption of ferrous iron preparations. Sustained-release preparations, which are expensive, are not more effective than standard formulations of iron, and the bioavailability is not greater. The administration of iron parenterally is justified if oral therapy has failed, or when patients are genuinely precluded from taking oral therapy. The rate of haemoglobin regeneration is not significantly faster when intramuscular or intravenous iron is used instead of the oral forms.

When parenteral therapy is required, intravenous administration is preferred, as absorption of iron from intramuscular sites may be variable.

ADVERSE EFFECTS OF ORAL THERAPY

The main adverse effects experienced with oral iron are those of *gastrointestinal intolerance*, which are described in approximately 20%–30% of patients. It has been suggested that many of the gastrointestinal effects experienced with oral iron are psychological, but this is not necessarily the case. Iron salts have astringent and locally irritative effects on the gastrointestinal mucosa, and the commonest symptoms of nausea and epigastric discomfort are dose-related and ascribed to a high local concentration of free iron. Oral doses in excess of 150 mg of iron a day are likely to make most patients unwell. Constipation and diarrhoea are less commonly dose-related. Adverse bowel symptoms may respond to reduction of dose, or to changing to an alternative preparation, as considerable individual variation exists in patients' response to the various formulations. Administration of iron with meals may reduce these effects, but food is also likely to diminish absorption.

The comparatively better tolerance of slow-release

iron medications may reflect the smaller amounts of iron available with these formulations. Higher concentrations of free iron are released in the small intestine, and correspondingly less in the stomach and duodenum. Upper gastrointestinal symptoms may be less than with standard preparations, but the incidence of constipation and diarrhoea is likely to be the same.

Acute hypersensitivity reactions to oral iron are very rare, and there is no evidence that hypersensitivity to parenteral iron is connected with gastrointestinal intolerance to oral preparations.

There are a few reports of *intestinal ulceration and perforation* due to high concentrations of locally released iron from delayed release preparations, and of intestinal obstruction in patients with bowel strictures (such as in Crohn's disease) due to impaction of unabsorbed matrices of capsules.

In children iron-containing syrups may *stain the teeth* reversibly; the discolouration may persist for weeks or months.

HAZARDS OF
PARENTERAL THERAPY

When parenteral iron is administered concomitantly with oral iron there is a danger that iron overload may be produced as transferrin may already be saturated, and the unbound iron may cause an acute toxic reaction.

The most important, although rare, complication of parenteral iron therapy is an *acute hypersensitivity reaction* which is characterised by collapse, hypotension, respiratory distress, cyanosis, facial oedema and urticaria. Anaphylactoid purpura has been reported. While prediction of this response is not possible, a previous sensitivity to iron (gastrointestinal intolerance not included) may alert the physician to the possibility.

A syndrome of painful lymphadenopathy, lumbosacral pain, high fever, tachycardia, markedly raised ESR, and a transient shock-like state has been described with parenteral iron therapy. The mechanism is not known; it may be an immune complex disease, and serum gamma globulins are sometimes raised.

Non-specific arthralgia has been described with parenteral iron therapy.

The administration of intravenous iron has been associated with *acute exacerbation of rheumatoid arthritis*, with fever and a flare-up of joint symptoms. This effect is peculiar to intravenous iron and to deposition of high concentrations of iron in synovium and joint fluid, suggesting local sensitivity, although the precise mechanism is not understood.

The relationship of intramuscular iron dextran (Imferon) and soft tissue sarcomas, which has been debated for years, is not supported by epidemiological evidence in humans.

IRON SUPPLEMENTS

Supplements for prophylactic purposes are given to prevent iron deficiency in pregnancy. The normal dose in pregnancy is 100 mg daily. No other justification exists for supplemental or prophylactic iron, and the practice may be unsafe. There is a risk of iron overload, and the correct diagnosis of other anaemias may be obscured.

FURTHER READING

Bothwell TH et al. (eds) (1979) Iron metabolism in man. Oxford, Blackwell
British National Formulary (1981) No 2. The British Medical Association and the Pharmaceutical Society of Great Britain, London, p 227
Kerr DNS (1958) Gastrointestinal intolerance to oral iron preparations. Lancet II:489
Reddy PS, Lewis M (1969) Adverse effects of intravenous iron-dextran in rheumatoid arthritis. Arthritis Rheum 12:454

2.11 Diabetes Mellitus

The large majority of insulin-dependent diabetics can be controlled satisfactorily with one of the standard forms of insulin. Perfect normoglycaemia and aglycosuria cannot be achieved in diabetic patients with insulin and neither should they be strived for. Most insulin still available is a mixture of beef and pork pancreatic extract or monospecies of beef or pork material. In mixed-species insulin about 60%–75% is the beef component insulin.

There is good evidence that diabetic control lessens chronic complications of the disease which are caused by microvascular injury, for example retinopathy. Good diabetic control is *thought* to improve the outcome in patients with diabetic neuropathy and cataract. The development of these complications is related to the duration and severity of the hyperglycaemia. It is not known whether diabetic control influences atheromatous disease.

Single-peak insulins produced and distributed in North America, Europe and elsewhere are greater than 98% pure.

INSULIN ALLERGY

Local reactions to insulin at the site of injection are common. Stinging, burning or itching may occur within an hour or two, and violaceous discoloration of the area may persist for several days. Such reactions usually develop in the first few weeks of therapy and then subside gradually. Rarely they may persist. Infrequently, generalised allergic reactions such as urticaria, pruritus and angioedema accompany local reactions. Anaphylactic reactions to insulin are rare.

Allergy to insulin has been attributed to protein contaminants. However, studies with single-peak beef and pork insulins suggest that these have few immunological advantages over less purified standard insulin. Immunoglobin E has been identified as the reaginic antibody, and this appears to be directed against the insulin molecule itself. Concentrations of circulating IgE correlate reasonably well with the clinical state. A history of prior intermittent use of insulin is present in many of these individuals.

The basis of management of these complications is the change to a less antigenic insulin preparation. Pork insulin is closer than beef to human insulin in its chemical composition, and is useful at times in reducing the allergic reactions seen with mixed forms. With insulin zinc preparations the possibility of a local response to zinc may be excluded by using an alternative preparation. Severe cases of insulin hypersensitivity may necessitate rapid insulin desensitisation. Once this has been achieved it is important that therapy should not be interrupted.

Only a few reports have been published of systemic allergic reactions to monocomponent insulins.

The use of purified insulin may necessitate a reduction in dosage, in most cases of the order of 20% −30%. However, some patients require no change in dosage and others may need higher doses of purified than of less purified insulin. It has yet to be demonstrated that a reduction in the immunogenic activity of insulin is of clinical benefit with respect to the long-term complications of diabetes mellitus.

INSULIN LIPOATROPHY AND LIPOHYPERTROPHY

Atrophy of subcutaneous fat tissue at the site of injection is a not uncommon complication of insulin therapy, particularly in children and young women. It is harmless, but causes concern because of the cosmetic effects it produces. The estimated incidence is 5%–10% but it appears to be less frequent with the more purified insulins. It may be due to substances in the older forms with a lipolytic or lipid-mobilising effect.

Injection of monocomponent insulin directly into affected areas frequently dramatically improves lipoatrophy, normally over a period of 2–4 weeks. Not all experience has indicated this, however, and some observers have reported that lipoatrophy will not respond in patients with co-existent local insulin allergy until the latter has been controlled.

Hypertrophy of subcutaneous fat in sites of insulin injection is seen more commonly in adult males than in females. It may be related to repeated injection at the same site. The incidence is low, and rotation of injection sites reduces the possibility of it developing. Injection of newer forms of insulin into hypertrophied areas has not resulted in improvement.

INSULIN RESISTANCE

This is defined as an insulin requirement of at least 200 units daily over a sustained period of time in the absence of infection, acidosis or coma, or alternatively as a subnormal response to standard amounts of insulin. The natural history of insulin resistance is broadly as follows: 50% of patients develop it within 1 year of the onset of diabetes mellitus; the duration in two-thirds of patients is under 6 months, and in one-quarter of patients the duration is greater than 1 year. Rarely, the resistance persists for years. The daily insulin requirement in resistant patients is usually under 500 units; in approximately one-third of patients it exceeds 1000 units.

Theoretically, pathogenic mechanisms of insulin resistance exist at the pre-receptor, receptor and post-receptor levels. Two syndromes are recognised: type A and type B. In the type A syndrome there appears to be a primary receptor defect. Teenage girls are characteristically affected and the features are of elevated plasma insulin and a requirement for large doses of exogenous insulin. A marked decrease in insulin receptor concentration on circulating monocytes has been demonstrated in this group. Clinical characteristics include acanthosis nigricans, hirsutism, polycystic ovaries, amenorrhoea and mildly elevated plasma testosterone concentrations. In the type B syndrome an immunoglobin is present in the plasma that competitively inhibits insulin binding to its receptor. No increase in receptor concentration can be effected by food restriction.

The first line of management is to change the species of insulin being used to pure beef or preferably pure pork insulin. This is likely to bring about a 50% reduction in insulin requirement. Monocomponent insulins may be of value in patients who have developed antibodies to standard insulin. Sulphated insulin is less antigenic than bovine or porcine forms, and it combines less avidly with antibodies. At the same time sulphation reduces the biological activity. Sulphated insulin is likely to be immediately effective in a substantial proportion of insulin-resistant diabetics. With high-dose corticosteroid therapy a 75% success rate has been reported in patients who have failed to respond to other measures, but the onset of response may be delayed and there are the hazards of steroid therapy in a diabetic.

There is a danger of hypoglycaemia at the onset of remission brought about by any of these measures.

INSULIN
HYPOGLYCAEMIC
REACTIONS

These are referred to in the section on drugs and the elderly (see p. 144).

THE SOMOGYI EFFECT

Biochemical hypoglycaemia at night may be followed by a heavy glycosuria in the morning (a "glycosuric tide"), contributing to unstable control. This phenomenon of "hypoglycaemia begetting hyperglycaemia" is the Somogyi effect (see Fig. 2.7). Although the phenomenon is probably an over-emphasised cause of hyperglycaemia (which is usually due to excessive carbohydrate intake), it is nevertheless important that it does not escape detection. Patients exhibiting the effect are usually non-obese and many have a history of ketoacidosis.

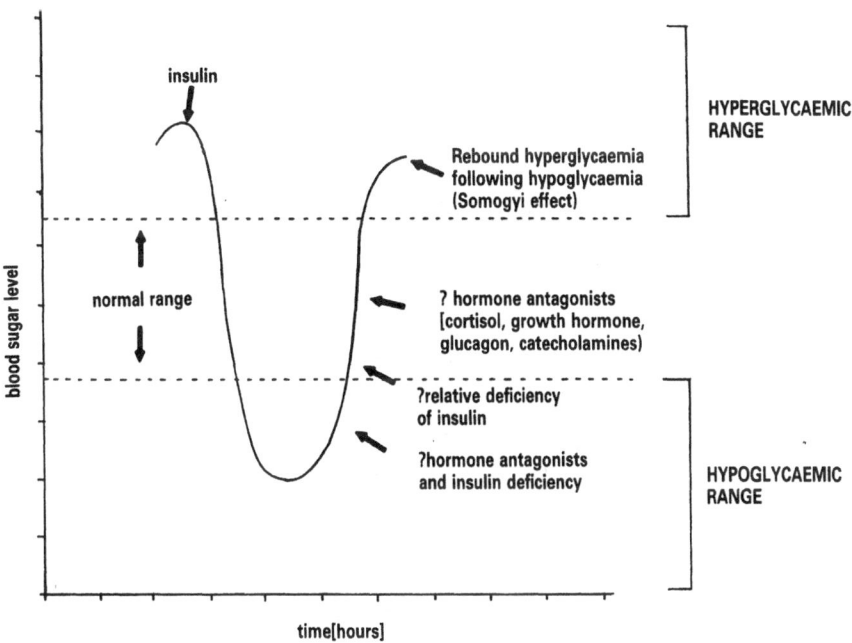

Fig. 2.7. Responses to insulin-induced hypoglycaemia and the Somogyi effect.

Hypoglycaemia at night is typically symptomless and may persist for hours. It may show itself as fits, which are easily mistaken for idiopathic epilepsy, or as mental dullness and depression lasting through the day.

Hypoglycaemia stimulates the release of insulin antagonists, cortisol, growth hormone, glucagon and catecholamines. The result of their concerted actions is increased glucose production and diminished utilisation. Early changes in blood glucose in response to hypoglycaemia are likely to be primarily due to reduction in free insulin, and this is probably a major factor in the hyperglycaemic response to hypoglycaemia. The net effect is an overshoot of blood glucose.

The Somogyi effect may be diagnosable only by measuring blood glucose in the early hours of the morning, and its control may require constant insulin delivery in the night if modification of insulin dosage is not successful.

BETA-ADRENORECEPTOR BLOCKING DRUGS AND BLOOD SUGAR CONTROL

Catecholamines participate in the reaction to hypoglycaemia and metabolic recovery from it. β-Adrenoreceptor blocking drugs might influence the response to insulin-induced hypoglycaemia. However, the incidence of loss of consciousness from hypoglycaemia does not appear to be greater in insulin-treated diabetics taking β-blockers compared with matched controls, and it may be concluded that this complication is rare. The principal objection to β-blockers in insulin-treated diabetics is that they might reduce or eliminate the warning symptoms of hypoglycaemia which are mediated by adrenergic stimulation. This is unlikely to be related to the dose of β-blocker. The rate of fall of blood glucose is not affected by β-blocker therapy, and likewise the rate of recovery. There is no evidence that selective β-blockers are less hazardous than non-selective agents in the diabetic patient. It can probably be concluded that, used skillfully, β-blocking drugs are safe for use in insulin-treated diabetics, and that it is unnecessary to deny diabetics the therapeutic benefit of these agents when they are needed.

SULPHONYLUREAS

Diet and reduction of excess weight are the foundations of initial therapy of the patient with adult-onset non-ketotic diabetes mellitus. Only when the condition cannot be adequately controlled by these measures (and, in the judgement of many physicians, when insulin is precluded because of patient unwillingness, poor adherence to injection regimen, physical disabilities such as poor vision and unsteady hand, insulin allergy, employment requirements, and other similar factors) is oral antidiabetic therapy advised. The sulphonylureas are usually the first line in this approach.

Contraindications to the use of sulphonylurea agents are severe diabetes mellitus, pregnancy, major surgery, severe stress such as acute trauma, severe infection, and renal or hepatic failure which might interfere with their metabolism or excretion.

The overall incidence of adverse effects is estimated at 3%–6% of patients. The most serious have been white cell depression and bone marrow aplasia. This appears to be a hypersensitivity response, and patients who have experienced a previous severe reaction should not be exposed to the risk of repeat administration.

Sulphonylurea-induced hypoglycaemia, particularly that caused by the long-acting chlorpropamide, may be severe and prolonged. Patients with renal or hepatic impairment and the elderly are at particular risk. Insidious development of renal failure leading to drug accumulation, concurrent use of other drugs which interfere with elimination, or displacement from plasma protein binding sites by phenylbutazone, oral anticoagulants or salicylates may contribute to this problem. Other sulphonylureas which are excreted unchanged or as pharmacologically active metabolites, such as acetohexamide and tolazamide (see Table 2.9) should be avoided in renal failure, and preference should be given to a drug such as tolbutamide which is fully metabolised in the liver to inactive metabolites. Drugs which do not rely on hepatic metabolism, such as chlorpropamide, are indicated in patients with hepatic failure.

Table 2.9. Sulphonylureas used in the treatment of diabetes mellitus (based on Editorial 1981)

Drug	Time to maximum plasma concentration of parent drug (h)	Plasma elimination half-life of parent drug (h)	Form excreted by kidneys
Acetohexamide	?	2–5	Active metabolites
Chlorpropamide	2–4	36	Parent drug
Glibenclamide	2–5	6	Inactive metabolites
Glibornuride	2–4	8	Inactive metabolites
Gliclazide	2	12	Inactive metabolites
Glipizide	1–2	2.5–4	Inactive metabolites
Gliquidone	2–3	1.5	Inactive metabolites
Glymidine	?	5–8	Active metabolites
Tolazamide	4–8	8	Active metabolites
Tolbutamide	4–6	5–8	Inactive metabolites

About three out of ten patients selected for oral hypoglycaemic therapy with sulphonylureas fail to respond *ab initio*. The most likely reason is that in such cases decompensated β-cells cannot be stimulated to release insulin. Such inadequate response from the start of therapy is referred to as primary failure. It may be related to the initial severity of the diabetes, failed compliance, and the adequacy of dietary control. After a remission induced by insulin subsequent treatment by diet and oral agents may be possible.

Relapse after convincing initial success is termed secondary failure. Failure rates vary with the criteria employed and they increase with duration of treatment. An estimated 5% of treated patients may be expected to relapse per year. Changing to a different oral antidiabetic agent may sometimes re-establish control. Not uncommonly secondary failure with one sulphonylurea may be reversed by changing to a different sulphonylurea. Little useful purpose is served in the case of either primary or secondary failure by increasing the dose of sulphonylurea above the maximum recommended. Indeed, tolbutamide in excessive dosage may raise rather than lower the blood sugar level.

The basis for secondary failure is likely to be inadequate release of insulin by the β-cells in response to the sulphonylurea, although other factors may be important as well. The addition of a biguanide may be effective in secondary failure; if not, insulin is required without delay.

It is very difficult to ascertain whether the use of the sulphonylureas has affected the incidence of occlusive arterial disease in diabetic patients. Of a number of studies directed at the influence of oral antidiabetic therapy on macro- and micro-angiopathy in diabetic patients, the University Group Diabetes Programme in the United States of America came to the alarming conclusions that fixed doses of tolbutamide or phenformin for over 5 years were associated with an increased death rate from all causes, and from cardiovascular diseases. No clear benefit was secured by either agent with non-fatal events complicating diabetes mellitus such as retinopathy, neuropathy and blindness. These findings are controversial; the United States Food and Drug Administration has not ruled finally on them, and they have been contested by workers elsewhere.

LACTIC ACIDOSIS

Lactic acidosis has been consistently reported with phenformin, although the true incidence of the association is not known. It is uncommon, but the mortality is high. In half the cases attributed to phenformin the patients have died. For this reason it is most important that patients who are at special risk should be identified. The onset of lactic acidosis is probably directly related to excessive accumulation of phenformin in the plasma and tissues, and patients with renal insufficiency, including transient disturbances of renal function, are particularly liable to develop this complication. Phenformin-induced lactic acidosis has also been described in association with cirrhosis and other forms of liver disease, perhaps because of the impaired capacity of the liver in such circumstances to remove excess lactate from the circulation. Renal failure itself, in the absence of phenformin therapy, is not a recognised cause of lactic acidosis. About half the cases of phenformin lactic acidosis arise during the first one to two months of treatment. The remainder may occur at any time thereafter and the onset may be quite unpredictable.

Other factors might contribute to lactic acidosis in diabetic patients receiving this group of agents, namely, prolonged fasting, severe dehydration due to persistent vomiting, and acute infections such as pyelonephritis and bronchopneumonia.

Early recognition of the condition is essential if there is to be a reasonable hope of successful treatment. Patients are acutely ill and dyspnoeic. Hyperventilation is usual but not always obvious. Vomiting and abdominal pain are common. The state of consciousness may be normal at first, progressing to mild drowsiness and eventually to coma. The blood pressure is maintained at first and the extremities well perfused, but if the condition remains untreated or fails to respond to treatment, shock develops after a few hours.

Most cases of phenformin-related lactic acidosis have been described in diabetics, but there are reports of the complication developing in non-diabetics having taken large doses of the drug for other purposes.

The biochemical features are a severe metabolic acidosis in which the arterial pH is commonly less than 7.0. Measurement of the blood lactate (normal concentration 0.4–1.3 mmol/l) is the surest way of confirming the diagnosis, although this laboratory investigation is only available in a limited number of centres. An anion gap (determined by subtracting the sum of the plasma chloride and bicarbonate concentrations from the sodium concentration; the normal difference being 12–15 mEq/l, representing unmeasured anions, including albumin, in the plasma) greater than 25 mEq/l is highly suggestive of the condition, provided the elevation of anion gap cannot be accounted for by ketone bodies, salicylates or uraemia. In some cases the anion gap may be marginal and the diagnosis correspondingly more difficult. Ketoacidosis and lactic acidosis can coexist, particularly in patients with alcoholic ketosis or diabetic ketoacidosis in whom there is poor tissue perfusion. In the absence of lactate measurements these combinations may be difficult to detect.

Thus, precipitous development of unexplained severe hyperventilation, the presence of an increased anion gap, and evidence of metabolic acidosis in a critically ill patient with compromised cardiovascular function in the absence of ketoacidosis, chronic renal failure or both will permit a firm diagnosis in patients receiving the drug.

The problem of biguanide-related lactic acidosis can be minimised by avoiding this group of agents (phenformin, metformin, and buformin) in patients with renal disease, cardiac failure or hepatic impairment. As a general rule the dose of phenformin should be kept to a minimum, not exceeding 100 mg/d, and that of metformin at less than 2 g daily. These drugs should always be withdrawn when patients develop serious intercurrent illnesses, including infections, myocardial infarction and other conditions likely to cause hypotensive shock. In such cases hypoglycaemia should be controlled with insulin. Despite these numerous restrictions there is still a place for biguanide treatment after dieting and sulphonylureas have failed, and in the very obese diabetic patient. The evidence is substantial that metformin is safer than phenformin in respect of this complication, and metformin is now the biguanide of choice. Buformin appears to occupy an intermediate position.

CHLORPROPAMIDE-
ALCOHOL FLUSH

Many diabetics treated with chlorpropamide show facial flushing after taking a small quantity of alcohol. It has been suggested that this effect may have a genetic basis, and that it might be a disulfiram-like reaction, mediated by acetaldehyde. There is indeed some evidence that chlorpropamide may inhibit aldehyde dehydrogenase. The true incidence is probably low, and does not appear to have relevance to the management of the majority of patients with non-insulin-dependent diabetes mellitus.

FURTHER READING

Barnett AH (1981) Chlorpropamide-alcohol interaction. Br Med J 283:939
Barnett AH et al. (1980) Insulin treated diabetics given beta-adrenergic blocking agents. Br Med J 280:976
Cohen RD (1978) Drugs and lactic acidosis. Adverse Drug Reaction Bull No 70:248
Editorial (1977) Biguanides, selection. Br Med J IV:1436
Editorial (1980) Diabetic control at night. Lancet II:279
Editorial (1981) Sulphonylurea selection in diabetes mellitus. Drug Ther Bull 19:49
Flier FS et al. (1979) Insulin resistance. N Engl J Med 300:413
Gale EAM et al. (1980) In search of the Somogyi effect. Lancet II:279
Gorden P (1977) Insulin resistance. In: Crepaldi G et al. (eds) Diabetes, obesity and hyperlipidemias. Academic Press, London, p 128
Kilo C et al. (1980) The Achilles heel of the U.G.D.P. JAMA 243:450
Kreisberg RA (1980) Lactate homeostasis and lactic acidosis. Ann Intern Med 92:227
Reaven GM (1980) Insulin allergy. In: Podolsky S (ed) Clinical diabetes. Modern management. Appleton Century Crofts, New York, p 114
Reeves WG et al. (1980) Insulin lipoatrophy and lipohypertrophy. Br Med J 280:1500
Wright AD (1979) Beta-adrenoreceptor blocking drugs and blood sugar control in diabetes mellitus. Br Med J I:159

2.12 Gout

The aims in the treatment of gout are (1) to terminate the acute attack as promptly as possible; (2) to prevent recurrences of acute gouty arthritis; (3) to prevent or reverse complications of the disease resulting from deposition of monosodium urate crystals in joints, kidneys and other sites; (4) to prevent or reverse associated features such as obesity, hypertriglyceridaemia, or hypertension; and (5) to prevent formation of uric acid kidney stones.

Drug therapy is central to most of these, and the following safety issues are of relevance.

COLCHICINE

Colchicine is an anti-inflammatory agent which achieves high levels in the leucocytes, and is said to inhibit the migration of granulocytes into the inflamed area, although its action in acute gout is almost certainly due to other pharmacological effects in addition.

The common adverse effects of the drug on the gastrointestinal tract in overdosage, namely, nausea, vomiting, diarrhoea and abdominal pain, are the earliest signs of toxicity, and cessation of the drug is necessary as soon as they occur. Individual variation exists in the toxic response to colchicine, and it may be that adverse effects are unavoidable in a particular patient during colchicine medication. Patients are often consistent in their responses to the drug, and therefore it may be possible by rating the threshold of toxicity to minimise or avoid adverse effects during subsequent courses of therapy. When given intravenously colchicine is as effective as when administered orally; the rate of onset may be faster, and the gastrointestinal side-effects may be avoided.

In severe colchicine toxicity profuse watery diarrhoea and haemorrhagic gastroenteritis may develop. Considerable fluid, electrolyte and plasma losses from the bowel may occur. Shock, renal damage, muscular depression and ascending paralysis of the central nervous system resulting in respiratory arrest have been reported.

Considerable caution is required in aged or feeble patients, and in patients with cardiac, renal or gastrointestinal disease.

INDOMETHACIN

See the section on the non-steroidal anti-inflammatory agents, p. 25.

Indomethacin is potentially hazardous in patients whose renal function is already impaired. Transient deterioration, possibly with hyperkalaemia, may develop. This seems to be due to a combination of impairment of water and sodium excretion at the proximal tubule, reduction of glomerular filtration, and alteration of renal haemodynamic autoregulation, as a result of the drug's action as inhibitor of prostaglandin synthetase activity. (In general, prostaglandin synthetase inhibitors should probably be avoided in patients with severe renal ischaemia with high levels of intrarenal vasoconstrictors.)

For these reasons indomethacin should be used with special caution in patients with pre-existing uraemia or congestive cardiac failure. The possibility of deterioration in renal status warrants careful monitoring of urinary output and renal function in patients who may be at risk.

On balance, although the side-effects of indomethacin when used in acute gout may be high, it is generally better tolerated than colchicine, and arguably is the treatment of choice in acute gouty arthritis.

Prolonged administration of indomethacin has been associated rarely with depression of the bone marrow, presenting as aplastic anaemia, agranulocytosis, or thrombocytopenia.

URICOSURIC AGENTS

The uricosuric drugs (notably probenecid and sulphinpyrazone) are used in chronic gout. In most patients ($\pm$ 70%) they cause uric acid to be excreted at a rate sufficient to exceed that of formation, thus lowering the plasma uric acid concentration. Prolonged oral administration to patients with tophaceous gout approximately doubles the daily urinary excretion of urates.

The uricosuric agents depend for their efficacy on sound renal function. They lose their effectiveness as creatinine clearance falls, becoming completely ineffective when clearance is less than 30 ml/min. Aspirin in any dose competitively blocks the uricosuric effect of probenecid and sulphinpyrazone.

On initiation of uricosuric therapy a negative urate balance is created; the serum urate falls, and urinary uric acid excretion may be considerably elevated above pre-treatment levels. This is transient and usually only lasts days, but may lead in a few patients to the development of renal calculi.

In order to minimise the risk the initial doses of uricosuric agents should be low. The hazard of acute uric acid nephropathy may be reduced by promoting the flow of a large volume of urine and alkalinising the urine with orally administered sodium bicarbonate.

The ideal candidate for uricosuric agents is under 60 years of age, has normal renal function, a uric acid excretion of less than 700 mg per day, and does not give a history of renal stones.

Sulphinpyrazone is a metabolite of phenylbutazone, without the anti-inflammatory activity of the latter. The two drugs share a similar toxic profile: gastrointestinal intolerance, bone marrow depression with thrombocytopenia and granulocytopenia, potentially serious redistributional interaction with warfarin sodium and an anti-natriuretic effect with fluid retention and possible deterioration of pre-existent cardiac failure.

ALLOPURINOL

Allopurinol is a xanthine oxidase inhibitor. It controls hyperuricaemia by inhibition of the terminal steps in uric acid biosynthesis. Its association with hypersensitivity reactions is referred to in the section on drug injury. An allopurinol hypersensitivity syndrome manifested by a prolonged illness with fever, cutaneous reaction, eosinophilia, hepatitis and renal failure is recognised. Impaired renal function is a special risk factor in the pathogenesis of hypersensitivity responses to allopurinol (see p. 171).

In blocking the conversion of xanthines to uric acid, allopurinol may cause an acute redistribution of the uric acid pool at the time of initiation of treatment. This may precipitate an attack of gout. Colchicine has been used with allopurinol to prevent this, although its efficacy has not been established beyond doubt.

Allopurinol potentiates the therapeutic and toxic effects of azathioprine and 6-mercaptopurine. The metabolism of these antimetabolites is altered in the same way as that of naturally occurring pyrimidines. The standard dose of 6-mercaptopurine should be reduced to a quarter when allopurinol is given at the same time.

The indications for using allopurinol in preference
to a uricosuric drug include (i) a particularly high
urinary uric acid secretion (e.g. greater than 700
mg/d); (ii) impaired renal function; (iii) tophaceous
gout, regardless of renal function; (iv) uric acid
nephrolithiasis; and (v) gout not controlled by
uricosuric agents because of ineffectiveness or
intolerance.

FURTHER READING

Baumelou A et al. (1980) Acute renal failure during indomethacin treatment. Acad Rev Calif
Acad Periodontol US Sect 9:3611
Flower RJ et al. (1980) Colchicine. In: Gilman AG, Goodman LS, Gilman A (eds) The pharmaco-
logical basis of therapeutics, 6th edn. Macmillan, New York, p 718
Lupton GP, Odom RB (1979) Allopurinol hypersensitivity syndrome. J Am Acad Dermatol 1:365

2.13 Myasthenia Gravis

Two therapeutic approaches are used to overcome the block of neuromuscular transmission in myasthenia gravis: agents with anticholinesterase
action are administered to increase and prolong activity of acetylcholine at
the myoneural junction; in more severe forms corticosteroids or thymectomy
directed at suppressing the immune response may be employed, often in
combination with anticholinesterases.

ANTICHOLINESTERASES   Anticholinesterases act by inhibiting acetylcholin-
esterase activity at the neuromuscular end-plate,
and by direct end-plate stimulation. It is not clear
how much of the effect is attributable to the latter.
They have in common an ammonium structure
which limits their penetration of cell membranes
(particularly the quaternary ammonium
compounds neostigmine bromide and pyridostigmine). Access to the brain of these quaternary
ammonium compounds is limited, which minimises their potential for adverse central nervous
system effects. Physostigmine, which has a tertiary
ammonium structure, has considerable activity in
the nervous system. Individual differences exist in
absorption, metabolism and elimination; in the
case of pyridostigmine, inactivation of which

commences in the gut wall, differences may be seven-fold. These account for the discrepancies in doses and dose frequency that may be required to control patients and indicate the necessity for individualisation of treatment in each case. Furthermore, dose requirements may vary in an individual from day to day, depending upon variables such as physical or emotional stress, menstruation, constipation and intercurrent infections.

Not uncommonly in myasthenia gravis toxic doses of anticholinesterases are inadvertently administered. Excessive amounts are sometimes given in a futile attempt at complete control of symptoms, particularly extraocular muscle weakness.

It has been stated that neostigmine causes adverse effects more frequently than pyridostigmine or ambenonium chloride, but it is doubtful whether the therapeutic index differs since neostigmine also tends to be more effective in certain patients.

Ambenonium chloride is a bisquaternary ammonium salt. Its reputed advantage is a prolonged duration of action, but many physicians find that it has no real advantage over pyridostigmine and it is not widely employed in the treatment of myasthenia gravis. It is occasionally well tolerated by patients who have severe muscarinic side-effects with neostigmine or pyridostigmine.

In toxic doses anticholinesterases produce excessive stimulation of muscarinic receptor responses at autonomic effector organs and in the CNS, and stimulation followed by paralysis of nicotinic receptors in autonomic ganglia and skeletal muscle. Muscarinic effects include nausea, vomiting, diarrhoea, intestinal cramps, bradycardia, micturition, sweating, salivation, lacrimation and bronchial secretion. There may be hypotension. With gross overdosage neostigmine and pyridostigmine may enter the nervous system and cause agitation, mental clouding and ultimately coma. Nicotinic effects are muscle fasciculations, cramps and increased weakness ("cholinergic blockade").

A *cholinergic crisis* is caused by massive accumulation of acetylcholine at the myoneural junction. An acute emergency is created, requiring pulmonary support and atropine to alleviate muscarinic side-effects.

ATROPINE
Atropine has been advocated for routine use together with neostigmine, pyridostigmine and ambenonium to reduce muscarinic effects, thereby allowing larger doses to be employed. Failure to use atropine may in certain instances preclude the achievement of maximal muscle strength. On the other hand, the use of atropine in this way can mask muscarinic effects, allowing nicotinic side-effects including muscle weakness to build up. Judicious use of atropine is therefore essential.

When other diseases are present in association with myasthenia gravis, such as bronchial asthma, parkinsonism, peptic ulceration and various cardiac diseases, there may be a theoretical objection to the use of drugs with cholinergic activity.

CORTICOSTEROIDS
Patients with severe or life-threatening myasthenia, who have failed to respond to other measures, may respond to corticosteroids. It would be useful to identify those most likely to benefit from steroids. Despite a lack of controlled studies, it has been suggested that older patients, those with purely ocular disease, and patients with thymoma—particularly if it is invasive—are most likely to be helped.

A reduced requirement for anticholinesterases in patients treated with corticosteroids may manifest itself in increased muscarinic side-effects, although this is not always noticeable. The possibility of a reduced requirement for anticholinesterases during corticosteroid therapy has to be borne in mind. At the same time, discontinuation or rapid reduction of dosage of an anticholinesterase may result in acute deterioration. Even when there is a good response to steroids many patients require anticholinesterase therapy in addition to maintain optimal function.

A dramatic deterioration in muscle strength may develop early in steroid therapy in certain patients. This hazard seems to be greatest in severe myasthenia. (Not all authorities accept that there is greater risk of initial deterioration.) It is generally accepted that commencement of steroid therapy should be under careful control, ideally in hospital, with small doses being given, which are increased progressively. The minimum effective dose is sought once control is established. From time to time further attempts at dose reduction can be made.

Other side-effects of corticosteroids in myasthenia gravis include systemic effects such as cushingoid appearance, glucose intolerance and hypothalamic-pituitary-adrenal suppression.

A child or adolescent is at risk of growth impairment; in such patients it is preferable first to attempt to achieve remission by thymectomy. Patients with concomitant diseases, such as diabetes mellitus and peptic ulceration, in whom steroids may be hazardous are excluded from this treatment.

OTHER DRUGS AFFECTING THE MYONEURONAL JUNCTION

Various drugs affect neuromuscular transmission, although it is rarely of clinical importance in patients with normal function. Weakness has occurred in non-myasthenics receiving aminoglycoside antibiotics, colistin, polymyxin, quinidine and procainamide with very high levels present owing to renal disease, or when different agents with neuromuscular blocking activity have been used together. (Penicillin, chloramphenicol, erythromycin, the cephalosporins and vancomycin have not caused such problems.) Lincomycin and clindamycin have been linked with deterioration in myasthenia. In acute infectious illnesses in myasthenics various antibiotics are preferably avoided, but where there are cogent reasons for their use they are given with considerable caution. β-Blockers and lignocaine, although potentially hazardous, have been used effectively when carefully administered.

Many authors consider barbiturates and morphine to be contraindicated in the myasthenic patient. Any agent that may depress respiration could be dangerous. When necessary, these drugs can be used in standard dose provided monitoring and support is assured.

FURTHER READING

Aquilonius SM et al. (1980) Pharmacokinetics and oral bioavailability of pyridostigmine in man. Eur J Clin Pharmacol 18:423
Dawkins RL et al. (1981) Myasthenia gravis and D-penicillamine. J Rheumatol 8 [suppl 7]:169
Lisak RP, Barchi RL (1982) Myasthenia gravis. Saunders, Philadelphia

Mastaglia FL, Argov Z (1981) Drug-induced neuromuscular disorders in man. In: Walton, Sir
    John (ed) Disorders of voluntary muscle, 4th edn. Churchill Livingstone, Edinburgh, p 873
Rodat O et al. (1981) D-Penicillamine induced myasthenic syndromes in rheumatoid arthritis.
    Nouv Presse Med 10:1645
Seybold ME, Drachman DB (1974) Prednisone in myasthenia gravis. N Engl J Med 290:81

3 Patients at Special Risk

3.1 Pregnant Women

Drug Injury to the Fetus

The following principles, based on clinical and experimental findings, are directly relevant to the drug treatment of pregnant women:

1. Several expressions of effect on the fetus of a teratogen are possible:
   i) *No apparent damage.* A teratogen may need to act in a complementary fashion with genetic and environmental factors in causing fetal injury.
   ii) *Structural malformations.* These do not occur when a teratogen is administered prior to embryonic organ differentiation. At this stage all cells are alike, and if the agent is potent enough to kill or severely damage cells, they tend to be affected in like manner. Structural organ defects occur when groups of cells have differing susceptibilities and growth patterns.
   iii) *Growth retardation, long-term psychomotor and behavioural effects.* After the period of organogenesis less obvious abnormalities of fetal development may be noted, although teratogens such as warfarin sodium may cause abnormal structural effects at any stage during pregnancy.
   iv) *Fetal death.* An agent capable of causing fetal malformations also causes an increase in mortality. It seems that death and abnormal development are different degrees of reaction to the same noxious stimulus, depending upon the dose of the toxin.

2. In the case of many teratogens embryos are able to tolerate small doses without permanent change, thus exhibiting a "margin of tolerance". Each embryo has a threshold above which irreparable changes occur. This is the teratogenic zone. An increment in dose can result in fetal death. The threshold for malformations rises with advancing fetal age, as does the threshold for mortality.

3. Susceptibility to teratogens depends upon the genotype of the conceptus.

The relative effects of genetic and external influences which interact to produce a defect probably range from those that have major genetic causation to a minority that have predominant environmental causation.

4. At the "critical period" of organogenesis the highest frequency of anatomical defects is seen. In the human, organogenesis is between about the 4th and 12th weeks of fetal life.

5. Widely differing agents frequently produce similar defects, suggesting a common final expression of abnormality. Effects are not necessarily specific to the causative factor, be it ionising radiation, drug, chemical teratogen or nutritional deficiency.

6. Teratogenic influences acting directly on the fetus are determined by their degree of access to vulnerable tissues.

Ionising radiations reach the conceptus directly, but chemical teratogens are generally first modified by the maternal organism. Whether or not chemicals or their degradation products reach the fetus in significant concentrations depends upon dosage, absorption, concentration in maternal blood, and maternal excretion, detoxification or storage of the compound. The placenta is frequently not a barrier to foreign chemicals. Many molecules of small size (less than 600 molecular weight) and low ionic charge cross by simple diffusion, others by facilitated diffusion, active transport, pinocytosis or simple leakage. Lipophilic entities readily cross the placenta.

DRUG USAGE IN
PREGNANCY

The United Kingdom Medicines Commission recognised the following categories of drugs with respect to their safety in pregnancy:

  i) There is clinical or epidemiological evidence of safety of the drug in human pregnancy.

  ii) There is no, or inadequate, evidence of safety of the drug in human pregnancy but it has been in wide use for many years without apparent ill consequence, and animal studies have shown no hazard.

  iii) There is no, or inadequate, evidence of safety of the drug in human pregnancy.

  iv) It has been in wide use for many years without apparent ill consequence.

  v) There is evidence of harmful effects in pregnancy in animals.

  vi) There is epidemiological or other good evidence of hazard in human pregnancy.

  vii) There has been little human usage but there is no adverse animal evidence.

viii) There is no evidence as to safety in human pregnancy, nor is there evidence from animal work that it is free from hazard.

A practical classification of medicines according to teratogenic risk is given in Table 3.1.

Table 3.1. Classification of medicines according to teratogenic risk (based on Wilson 1979)

Known human teratogens	Suspected human teratogens	Possible human teratogens	Not believed to be teratogenic under normal conditions of use
Androgenic hormones	Alcohol	Anaesthetics	Barbiturates
Antineoplastic agents	Alkylating agents	Antibiotics	Marihuana
Folic acid antagonists	Anticonvulsants	Antihistamines	Narcotic analgesics
Organic mercury	Anorectic medicines	Antituberculous agents	
Thalidomide	Oral hypoglycaemic agents	Female sex hormones	
	Warfarin	Lithium carbonate	
		Quinine and other anti-malarials	
		Salicylates	
		Tricyclic antidepressants	

Drug Treatment of Important Medical Conditions in Pregnancy

The following *general guidelines* for the use of drugs in pregnancy have been put forward (see Rao and Arulappa, 1981):

1. No known dysmorphogenic drug should be given to women of child-bearing age unless a reliable form of contraception is being used.
2. No drug can be considered 100% safe to the fetus (including topical preparations).
3. A true indication must be present for the administration of any drug in pregnancy.
4. The effect on the fetus may not necessarily be the same as on the mother.

SEVERE VOMITING AND HYPEREMESIS GRAVIDARUM

Despite wide usage the effectiveness of antihistamines in prevention and treatment of nausea and vomiting of pregnancy has never been demonstrated in a controlled and objective fashion. An advisory committee of the United States Food and Drug Administration has recognised that whilst these agents are proven teratogens in some lower animals, available clinical data do not support an association in humans.

Antihistamines should be prescribed in pregnancy only if they are regarded as essential, in a dosage and duration of therapy that is kept to a minimum.

EPILEPSY

Approximately 0.5% of pregnant women are epileptic. Management presents major therapeutic problems.

The precise risk of congenital malformations among infants exposed in utero to anti-epileptic drugs is estimated to be two or three times greater than in the general population. The anomalies most often encountered are cleft palate, cleft lip and cardiac defects, particularly of the cardiac septum.

Most women who have epilepsy during pregnancy will have been identified prior to conception, and only a minority (less than 25%) have seizures confined to pregnancy ("gestational epilepsy"). If deterioration occurs in established epileptics it is likely to be in the first trimester. After delivery the previous seizure frequency is usually re-established.

An important reason for loss of seizure control during pregnancy is a decline in plasma anti-epileptic drug levels, despite a constant oral dose, which is due to altered pharmacokinetics. Plasma clearance of phenytoin and phenobarbitone increases and blood levels fall progressively during pregnancy, returning to pre-gravid levels after delivery.

In an epileptic woman contemplating pregnancy a drug regimen should be implemented that is based upon optimum seizure control, with fewest maternal side-effects, rather than on the risk of teratogenicity, which is small. Ideally single-drug therapy should be used, and this is most effectively achieved by maintaining plasma drug levels in the therapeutic range. As a general principle major changes in the anti-epileptic regimen should not be undertaken unless seizure control is poor. As pregnancy proceeds the doses required for maintenance may reach levels that would be toxic in the non-gravid state. The dose required to maintain a therapeutic level during pregnancy does not decline immediately post partum. High doses may be required for variable periods, reduction being planned according to plasma determinations.

The treatment of status epilepticus in the pregnant female is as for the non-pregnant state. Both the condition and its management have serious implications for the fetus.

RHEUMATIC
CONDITIONS

Aspirin is teratogenic in several mammalian species, but it has not been shown to cause human congenital malformations. However, mothers who take salicylates regularly during pregnancy may have a higher incidence of stillborn babies and infants with low birth weight. The teratogenicity potential of other prostaglandin synthetase inhibitors is not known.

Early exposure of the mammalian fetus to prostaglandin synthetase inhibitors has been shown in experimental animals to reduce the eventual number of pulmonary arterial vessels. Human maternal intake of indomethacin shortly before delivery has been associated with accelerated closure of the ductus arteriosus, which could result in potentially dangerous pulmonary hypertension in the newborn.

Salicylates compete with bilirubin for albumin binding sites, and if given towards the end of pregnancy they may heighten the danger of kernicterus. Salicylates in late pregnancy may interfere with platelet function, resulting in a bleeding tendency in the newborn.

TUBERCULOSIS

Experience has shown that the first-line drugs isoniazid and ethambutol have a reasonable margin of safety in pregnancy. Over 90% of pregnant women treated with them can expect to deliver normal infants.

Amongst all the antituberculotics streptomycin is associated with the highest incidence of malformations in the fetus. Approximately one in six newborns exposed in utero have some hearing loss or vestibular defect. The risk of this exists throughout gestation.

Isoniazid in combination with ethambutol and pyrazinamide is a widely accepted treatment of tuberculosis in pregnancy, provided the disease is not extensive. Streptomycin is added by most authorities during the first phase of treatment. If a more potent drug is necessary because of the extensive nature of the disease, rifampicin may be necessary. The teratogenic risk of rifampicin in humans has not been defined.

ULCERATIVE COLITIS

Women with active ulcerative colitis at the start of pregnancy have a smaller chance of producing a normal live baby than those in whom the disease is quiescent. (In the latter category the outcome of pregnancy appears to be similar to the overall population.) Acute exacerbations during pregnancy are generally mild and respond to treatment. Medical treatment of ulcerative colitis has not been shown to have deleterious effects on the fetus or newborn child.

ANTICOAGULATION

The coumarin anticoagulants (notably warfarin sodium) are human teratogens. The most striking and frequently reported anomalies in newborns are nasal hypoplasia and stippled epiphyses. Interference in the development of cartilage may account for these effects. Their approximate incidence is of the order of 20%.

Hydrocephalus, optic atrophy and mental retardation may develop in the fetus as a result of the use of warfarin at any time during pregnancy. The causal relationship of these defects with warfarin has yet to be proven.

Any anticoagulant administered during pregnancy creates a substantial risk of bleeding, and the use of heparin does not result in a better outcome than other agents. At best, two-thirds of infants will be normal at birth following use of heparin.

Because of the dangers of anticoagulants, and the inherent hazards of the indications for which they are prescribed, prevention of pregnancy in such patients may be preferable.

DEPRESSION

The Committee on Drugs of the American Academy of Pediatrics has reviewed the use of psychotropic agents in pregnancy. Consistent with the view that no medication should be prescribed for a pregnant woman unless it is necessary for her health or that of her child, the Committee recommended that where practical and consistent with controlling symptoms a woman should be withdrawn from psychotropic medication prior to conception.

When continued drug therapy is required the existing evidence provides no basis for selecting any particular psychotropic agent or agents.

Further Reading

American Academy of Pediatrics, Committee on Drugs (1979) Anticonvulsants and pregnancy. Pediatrics 63:331
American Academy of Pediatrics, Committee on Drugs (1982) Psychotropic drugs in pregnancy Pediatrics 69:241
Folb PI (1980) Prediction of the teratogenic potential of a new medicine. In: Safety of medicines: evaluation and prediction. Springer, Berlin Heidelberg New York, p 17
Fraser FC (1959) Causes of congenital malformations in man. J Chronic Dis 10:97
Girling DJ (1973) Tuberculosis in pregnancy. Tubercle 54:309
Girling DJ (1982) Tuberculosis in pregnancy. Drugs 23:56
Hall JG et al. (1980) Anticoagulation during pregnancy. Am J Med 68:122
Knight AH, Phind EG (1975) Epilepsy and pregnancy. Epilepsia 16:99
Levin D et al. (1978) Non-steroidal anti-inflammatory agents. J Pediatr 92:478
Manchester D et al. (1976) Non-steroidal anti-inflammatory agents. Am J Obstet Gynecol 126:467
Medicines Commission, United Kingdom (1977) Safety of drug usage during pregnancy. In: Annual report of the Medicines Commission, p 70
Montouris GD et al. (1979) The pregnant epileptic. Arch Neurol 36:601
Rao JM, Arulappu R (1981) Drug use in pregnancy. Drugs 22:409
Sadusk JF, Palmisano PA (1965) Report of an ad hoc advisory committee of the United States FDA on the teratogenicity of certain antihistamines. JAMA 194:139
Snider DE et al. (1980) Tuberculosis in pregnancy. Am Rev Respir Dis 122:65
Turner G, Collins E (1975) Non-steroidal anti-inflammatory agents. Lancet II:338
Willoughby CP, Truelove SC (1980) Ulcerative colitis and pregnancy. Gut 21:469
Wilson JG (1979) Handbook of teratology, vol 1. Plenum, New York

3.2 Breast-Feeding Mothers

Medicines taken by a lactating mother may pass into the milk. The following *general principles* may be of assistance in evaluating the likelihood and risks:

1. Few drugs are contraindicated in breast-feeding women, but supporting data for either proscriptions or permissive statements are often lacking.

2. Minute amounts of certain drugs may be toxic to neonates, owing to immature detoxification and metabolising systems.

3. Only essential drugs should be given to the nursing mother. Although only small amounts of drugs may be present, large volumes of milk are drunk

by the neonate. Usually, however, not more than 1%–2% of the total maternal dose is transferred by breast milk to the infant.

4. Difficulty arises with drugs for which there is no information available; comparison with a drug in a similar pharmacological group may be of some value, but even slight molecular changes can markedly affect excretion and toxicity. In such cases samples should be analysed if possible and the infant's progress carefully monitored.

5. Diuretics diminish milk flow and should be avoided if possible.

6. *Antituberculous agents*. Ethambutol in therapeutic doses does not have a toxic effect on the infant; isoniazid may be toxic and the infant should be carefully monitored; streptomycin is excreted in the breast milk; rifampicin has a low human milk to plasma ratio (0.2–0.6), but little can be said about its safety in the newborn. Mothers being treated for tuberculosis are normally advised to breast feed, as the small possibility of drug injury to the infant is offset by the advantages of proper feeding, particularly in a low socioeconomic population.

7. The concentration of the following drugs in breast milk is indicated in the breast milk:plasma ratios:

gentamicin	(2 : 1)
isoniazid	(1.6 : 1)
thiouracil	(1 : 1)
calcium	(1 : 1)
clindamycin	(1.7–1.1 : 1)
erythromycin	(4–5 : 1)
vitamin A	(1 : 1)

8. Ethanol is freely secreted into milk in concentrations slightly lower than those in the blood. There is no evidence that occasional moderate ingestion of alcohol by the mother is harmful to the infant. Intoxicated mothers, and chronic alcoholics who refuse to stop drinking, should not breast feed.

9. Bronchodilator drugs are often necessary, even if the patient is nursing her infant. Little information exists concerning the pharmacokinetics and potential risks to the infant of anti-asthmatic agents, with the exception of theophylline. It has been estimated that less than 10% of the mother's dose of theophylline will reach the infant, and adverse reactions in the infant are rare. As a rule, inhaled bronchodilators are not significantly absorbed, and lactating mothers should ideally be managed on inhalation therapy. The same applies to the use of inhaled beclomethasone, which is preferred to systemic corticosteroids.

The additive effect to theophylline of theobromine (present in chocolate) and caffeine, consumed in coffee, colas, tea and other foods, should be considered.

Additional information is provided in Table 3.2.

Table 3.2. Categories of risk of various drugs to the breast-fed infant (based on Berlin 1980)

Drugs incompatible with breast feeding[1]	Drugs which are possibly harmful to the infant[2]	Drugs which can affect milk production
Cytotoxic drugs	Antihistamines	Diuretics (decrease)
Immunosuppressive agents	Aspirin, in high doses	Oral contraceptives (inhibit)
Radiopharmaceuticals[3]	Carbimazole	Phenothiazines (increase)
	Central nervous system depressants	
	Chloramphenicol	
	Corticosteroids	
	Diuretics (potent, e.g. ethacrynic acid)	
	Ergot alkaloids[4]	
	Ethanol (large amounts)	
	Laxatives (potent forms such as cascara, aloes)	
	Lithium[5]	
	Narcotic analgesics	
	Propranolol[6]	
	Propylthiouracil[7]	
	Tetracyclines[8]	
	Warfarin[7]	

Numbers: refer to the following notes:

1. Breast feeding should be discontinued.

2. Close monitoring is essential; the advantages of use may outweigh the disadvantages. The benefit should outweigh the risk.

3. Milk should be counted for radioactivity before breast feeding is instituted.

4. Ergot is given to many nursing mothers in the first few days after delivery for uterine bleeding; no apparent side-effects are produced in infants as a result of such short-term exposure.

5. Hypotonia and cyanosis in the baby have been attributed to lithium in breast milk, but this is on the basis of limited clinical data.

6. Low maternal doses of propranolol (e.g. 250 mg/day or less) appear to be safe for the infant. However, close observations for evidence of bradycardia or hypoglycaemia should be carried out in these nursing infants. [See Bauer JH et al. (1979) Propranolol in human plasma and breast milk. Am J Cardiol 43:860]

7. Warfarin sodium and the antithyroid agent propylthiouracil, which have traditionally been regarded as contraindicated in lactating mothers, can probably be regarded as non-hazardous to the infants. [See Orme ML'E et al. (1977) May mothers given warfarin breast-feed their infants? Br Med J I:1564; Kampmann JP et al. (1980) Propylthiouracil in human milk. Lancet I:736]

8. Short courses of maternal tetracycline are probably not harmful.

It should be noted that the above classification does not mean that all other drugs are safe.

FURTHER READING

Berlin CM (1980) The excretion of drugs in human milk. In: Drugs and chemical risks to the fetus and newborn. Alan R Liss, New York, p 111

3.3 The Elderly

The significant physiological differences in the elderly compared with younger people may increase the potency and/or toxicity of drugs, and reduce their elimination by hepatic metabolism and renal excretion. Lean body mass and the plasma albumin are reduced in many old people; as a result of the former the volume of distribution of drugs which normally distribute to fatty tissues may be reduced, with a corresponding elevation in concentration in the central compartment. Drugs which are highly protein-bound are likely to concentrate in higher amounts in the serum in the unbound and active state when serum albumin is diminished. Drugs which are mainly excreted by the kidney may accumulate to dangerous levels if standard doses are administered to elderly patients.

Elimination of renally excreted drugs will be reduced in the older age group in proportion to reduction in renal function. For drugs with a high therapeutic ratio these differences are of little importance, but for digoxin and the aminoglycoside antibiotics dosage schedules must take into account the altered pharmacokinetics. For drugs that are not primarily excreted by the kidneys there is insufficient information on which to base dose recommendations in the elderly. Many elderly patients have multiple pathology, so that data obtained from healthy subjects may not be applicable.

Compliance in the elderly is often poor, particularly when they do not understand how and when to take the medicines prescribed, and when drug regimens are not straightforward. Elderly patients are often unaware of the hazards of suddenly discontinuing certain medicines.

There is little information regarding the value or otherwise of treating symptomless disease in the elderly, such as mild diabetes mellitus or hypertension. Excessive treatment of such conditions can make the situation worse.

Several drug-induced syndromes are recognised in the elderly:

DISINHIBITION
REACTIONS

Elderly patients may have uncontrollable outbursts of rage or paradoxical reactions of agitation and acute anxiety following the use of tranquillisers, sedatives, or ethanol. The benzodiazepines are the commonest identifiable cause of acute disinhibition reactions in this age group, perhaps because they are most widely used. This response is unexplained and not readily predictable, although it may be related to the underlying personality of the patient, and it may possibly be anticipated from a previous similar episode.

NEUROPSYCHIATRIC
SYNDROMES

In patients with limited cerebral reserve, central nervous system depressants (which may in this context include such agents as penicillin in high doses, isoniazid, and the non-steroidal anti-inflammatory agents) may cause impairment of recent memory, disorientation, restlessness, and impaired intellectual function and judgement.

Paranoia, hallucinations, incoherent speech, labile emotions and striking hyperactivity may develop, leading in the worst cases to dementia and coma. Drugs are an important cause of reversible dementia in this age group.

TRANQUILLISER DEPENDENCE

Reference has been made to the vicious cycle that may be established between sleeplessness and chronic benzodiazepine usage, withdrawal of which may result in a situation which itself is characterised by insomnia (see p. 44).

ANTICHOLINERGIC SYNDROME

The adverse CNS effects of drugs with anticholinergic activity (see pp. 48, 175) may be severe in the elderly. Toxic delirium or dementia, worsening of glaucoma, urinary retention and disturbances of temperature control are common in this age group.

HYPOGLYCAEMIC SYNDROMES

Several neuroglycopenic syndromes are recognised as a result of excessive insulin or oral hypoglycaemic therapy for diabetes mellitus. Symptoms are likely to be noted when the blood glucose level has fallen to 50% of its normal lower level; the elderly brain is especially jeopardised by the effects of hypoglycaemia.

An acute neuroglycopenic or insulin reaction (combined metabolic encephalopathy and catecholamine release) may occur in the elderly, as in other age groups. The sympathetic response associated with catecholamine release—tachycardia, palpitations, nervousness and tremor—may be absent in 50% of patients in this age group.

A subacute neuroglycopenic syndrome which may resemble chronic metabolic encephalopathy or chronic alcoholism is characterised by reversible poor task performance, decreased spontaneous motor activity, somnolence, intoxicated behaviour and lack of insight into mental deterioration.

Chronic neuroglycopenic brain injury may involve insidious personality change, defective memory, dementia and even the development of overt psychosis. The symptoms may be entirely psychiatric, and patients are sometimes inadvertently regarded as suffering from primary psychotic illness or dementia. Prolonged neuroglycopenia may result in irreversible brain damage.

The importance of avoiding excessive reduction of the blood sugar in elderly diabetics is emphasised by these various hazards of hypoglycaemia, particularly as this age group seems to adapt to higher than normal blood glucose levels.

OCULAR EFFECTS

Prolonged topical (or systemic) administration of corticosteroids may be complicated by the development of posterior subcapsular cataract or elevated intraocular pressure. The latter is likely to occur if a patient has chronic open-angle glaucoma or a family history of the condition.

Parasympathomimetic agents such as pilocarpine hydrochloride produce pupillary miosis and contraction of ciliary musculature, thus increasing aqueous humour outflow from the anterior chamber. They are commonly used in treating chronic open-angle glaucoma. Accommodative spasm with pilocarpine can occur in presbyopic individuals, and night vision may be reduced as a result of miotic pupils. Topical pilocarpine to the eye may cause systemic toxicity due to absorption, resulting in cholinergic effects.

Anticholinergic agents such as atropine and its congeners produce mydriasis and paralysis of the ciliary musculature (cycloplegia). They are used to treat anterior ocular inflammation (often following cataract extraction in elderly patients). Intraocular tension may rise, and in patients with glaucoma this may have dangerous consequences. Systemic absorption of atropine from the eye may occur, causing cholinergic manifestations including fever, disorientation and hallucinations.

SPECIAL ISSUES IN DRUG TREATMENT

Drug hazards in the treatment of disorders of the elderly, with recommendations and special precautions for their prevention, are listed in Table 3.3.

Table 3.3. Special issues in drug treatment of the elderly

Medical condition	Drugs	Hazards	Comments
Hypertension	Diuretics	The diuretic-induced combination of hyponatraemia, hypokalaemia, dehydration and hypotension in this age group may lead to the geriatric triad of immobility, incontinence and bedsores	It is not appropriate to attempt to achieve perfect control of blood pressure. Doses of anti-hypertensive agents should be titrated against patient response
	Antihypertensive agents	Postural hypotension is a special problem. Methyldopa and reserpine are potent causes of depression	
	β-Blockers	The adverse effects of β-blockers are likely to be accentuated	
Heart failure	Digitalis	Digitalis cardiotoxicity may not necessarily be associated with other toxic manifestations	A diuretic alone will usually suffice; digitalis therapy can often be discontinued without ill effect. When digitalis is required, a small daily or alternate-day dose (0.0625–0.125 mg) is usually enough
	Diuretics	Powerful diuretics such as frusemide can cause painful distension of the bladder in patients with urinary obstruction due to prostatic hypertrophy	
Insomnia	Benzodiazepines	Benzodiazepines may aggravate sleep disturbances (see text)	Short-term use of short-acting benzodiazepines may help. Chloral hydrate is safe and effective. Tricyclic antidepressants may be indicated in depressed patients
Anxiety	Phenothiazines	Phenothiazines taken long term may cause parkinsonism and tardive dyskinesia	
	Barbiturates	Barbiturates are unsatisfactory in the elderly, as they are likely to cause confusion, ataxia and unsteadiness	

Table 3.3. (*continued*)

Medical condition	Drugs	Hazards	Comments
Constipation	Laxatives	Liquid stools should be avoided as dehydration occurs easily. Liquid paraffin given repeatedly may permeate the bowel causing diarrhoea and even malabsorption, and it may be inhaled into the lungs if taken at night	Methylcellulose, glycerin suppositories and senna are safe
Depression	Monoamine oxidase inhibitors (MAOIs)	MAOIs are usually regarded as contraindicated in the elderly because they are so likely to cause hypomania and ataxia	
	Tricyclic anti-depressants	Elderly patients are often susceptible to the anticholinergic effects of these agents	Very small doses of tricyclic antidepressant are usually sufficient
Pain	Opiate alkaloids; morphine	The rate of elimination of opiates in elderly patients is considerably longer than in younger persons. Opiate toxicity is likely to develop in this age group due to reduced respiratory and cardiovascular reserve and possibly an increased tissue sensitivity. Anti-emetics given with morphine may aggravate respiratory depression The constipation caused by opiates may be a problem. Small doses of morphine do not often cause nausea and vomiting in the elderly	Opiates should only be given when absolutely necessary. For acute problems intravenous administration is preferred, as it avoids delayed absorption from intramuscular sites. Anti-emetics should be avoided unless the patient develops nausea. Signs of toxicity should be carefully sought. Morphine toxicity is treated with naloxone. Hypoventilation may recur after naloxone because its half-life is shorter than that of morphine

GUIDELINES

i) It is most important that an accurate diagnosis is made if drug therapy is to be helpful rather than useless or harmful. (For example, insomnia may be due to anxiety, depression, urinary frequency, cardiac failure or even low ambient temperature.)

ii) The use of a drug in an elderly patient has to be fully justified.

iii) Treatment in the elderly should not be continued for longer than necessary. Many diseases are episodic, and treatment should not be unduly extended in such cases.

iv) As few drugs as possible should be given, and there is a special need in this age category for regular review.

v) Placebos are useful but should be used with discrimination. It is important that the substance is truly inert.

vi) Compliance can be improved by ensuring that the patient understands how and when to take the medicine, by making the regime simple, and by providing visual aids for instruction of patients with poor eyesight. Containers should be easily handled (not "child-proof", as they are often elderly-proof as well). The help of relatives or other reliable persons should be enlisted when the patient seems unsure. Once-daily medication in liquid form is ideal.

vii) As a general rule, it is advisable to start with a dose of one-quarter to one-third of that recommended for adults, and gradually to work up from this. The half-life of elimination of drugs is likely to be of the order of 30% greater in this age group.

viii) New products should be tried with special caution.

ix) The hazards of suddenly withdrawing medicines should be appreciated.

FURTHER READING

Caradoc-Davies TH (1981) Opiate toxicity in elderly patients. Br Med J 283:905
Crooks J et al. (1976) Pharmocokinetics in the elderly. Clin Pharmacokinetics 1:280
Dangel ME, Havener WH (1981) Drugs in the ageing eye. Geriatrics 36:133
Ramsey LE, Tucker GT (1981) Drugs and the elderly. Br Med J 282:125
Williamson J (1980) Safe prescribing for the elderly. Geriatrics 35:32

3.4 Motor Vehicle Drivers

Several different groups of drugs prescribed for therapeutic purposes may be hazardous in combination when taken by persons who drive motor vehicles. This danger is shared by motorcyclists and workers operating complex machines, and by people who climb heights and may be at risk of falling. The precise effects of drug use on fine motor skills is not known, and it is possible that certain drugs may improve performance, while others cause a deterioration. The problem is confined to agents which act on the central nervous system.

Those drugs recognised as being prejudicial to safe driving are:

1. Antidepressants and tranquillisers.

2. Sleeping pills. In the case of hypnotics with a long elimination time from the body (e.g. more than 6–8 h) a motor vehicle driver may still be affected the morning after.

3. Drugs used against motion sickness and allergy. This applies particularly to the antihistamines. Combination drugs in this category may contain caffeine as a counter to drowsiness, but the caffeine is short-acting.

4. Pain-relieving agents of the central-acting type, which may be in combination with tranquillisers.

5. Central nervous system stimulants, many of which are distributed illegally.

6. Drugs used against epilepsy.

When these pharmacological agents are used by motor vehicle drivers, and others dependent upon fine motor skills, there is a risk of the driver becoming less alert, fatigued, drowsy, lethargic, faint, and less able to react spontaneously, with loss of judgement in traffic. Consequently there is a danger of the driver becoming prone to accident.

A further hazard is the interaction between medicines of these categories and ethanol. A critical blood alcohol concentration will impair sensory and motor function, reflex activity, concentration, insight, and the level of consciousness. When small doses of alcohol and another CNS-acting drug are taken together, a synergistic and undesirable effect may result.

It is very important that patients are aware of the risks that these drugs may present, particularly when ethanol is taken at the same time.

FURTHER READING

Ozorio P (1981) Danger in mixing psychotropics with driving. Publication No 71. Division of Public Information, World Health Organisation, Geneva

3.5 Porphyrics

Drugs are the most common of the identifiable precipitating factors in the acute porphyric attack in all three of the autosomal dominant inherited porphyrias, namely, acute intermittent porphyria (AIP), hereditary coproporphyria and variegate porphyria (VP). A wide variety of drugs may be responsible; barbiturates, the oral contraceptives and ethanol are the most common. Barbiturates are involved in over 50% of attacks, and in over 20% they are the only identifiable precipitants. Other agents frequently implicated are analgesics, sulphonamides, non-barbiturate hypnotics and sedatives, anticonvulsants and hormones. In symptomatic porphyria these are without deleterious effect.

A detailed list of medicines considered to be potentially hazardous in the hereditary porphyrias is presented in Table 3.4. Only those drugs which have been reported by three or more workers in the field to be associated with clinical exacerbations of porphyria have been included.

Table 3.4. Drugs in common use reported as dangerous in porphyria[1,2]

Antimicrobial agents:
    Dapsone
    Griseofulvin
    Pyrazinamide
    Sulphonamides
Anaesthetic agents:
    Barbiturates[3]
Anticonvulsants:[4]
    Barbiturates[3]
    Hydantoins (phenytoin, mesantoin)
    Carbamazepine
    Succinimides
Minor tranquillisers:[4]
    Glutethimide
    Methyprylone
    Meprobamate
Antidiabetic agents:
    Sulphonylureas
Antihypertensives:
    Alphamethyldopa
Narcotic analgesics:
    Pentazocine
Non-steroidal anti-inflammatory agents:
    Isopropyl antipyrine
    Amidopyrine
    Antipyrine
    Phenylbutazone
Miscellaneous:
    Ethanol
    Oral contraceptives[5]

Numbers refer to following notes:

1. This Table is not comprehensive, and because of the criteria applied for inclusion of items it is a conservative one (see text).

2. In AIP and VP drugs may precipitate acute attacks characterised by abdominal, neurological and neuropsychiatric manifestations, associated with a marked increase in urinary excretion of δ-aminolaevulinic acid (ALA) and porphobilinogen (PBG). The dangerous porphyrinogenic drugs may lead to profound quadriplegia and bulbar involvement, resulting, without adequate support, in respiratory failure and death.

3. When multiple barbiturate therapy has been given to porphyric patients attacks have generally been of a more severe nature than those precipitated by single drugs. On the other hand, exposure to thiopentone sodium and phenobarbitone, both of which are potentially dangerous, does not always lead to an acute attack. A past history of uneventful usage of a drug does not guarantee freedom from a devastating attack on subsequent exposure.

4. For "at-risk" subjects it is important that they are aware that over-the-counter medicines may contain tranquilliser or sedative agents which are potentially dangerous.

5. The oral contraceptives are amongst the most common of the identifiable precipitating factors in the acute porphyric attack.

CLINICAL GUIDELINES   The following information is important for the management of a patient with obscure abdominal pain which could be attributable to acute porphyria:

i) A past history of acute abdominal pain and/or paralysis, and whether these are known to be drug-related. Adverse sequelae of previous operations under anaesthesia are of particular relevance in this regard.

ii) Increased skin susceptibility to minor trauma which results in the development of blisters and erosions. The diagnosis of variegate porphyria is also suggested by the presence of luxuriant eyebrows associated with temporal hirsutism which may involve the face. In women particularly skin fragility may be minimal and the sun-exposed skin unblemished.

iii) Ehrlich's aldehyde test for porphobilinogen carried out in suspected porphyrics with acute symptoms and/or paralysis.

iv) Acute attacks and/or cutaneous involvement in the patient's immediate relatives, and biochemical investigation of urine and faeces for porphyrins.

MANAGEMENT OF AN ACUTE ATTACK

No specific therapy exists for the treatment of porphyria. Propranolol given early in the pre-paralytic phase of an acute attack is effective in reducing acute anxiety and controlling tachycardia and hypertension. The intractable abdominal pain requires powerful analgesia. Pethidine and dihydrocodeine may control pain, but morphine may be required. Vomiting can be controlled by promazine. The commonly observed neurosis and psychosis can be controlled with chlorpromazine or promazine, and seizures with diazepam. When constipation is severe, neostigmine may be helpful.

PREDICTION

One of the difficulties in the porphyrias is prediction of porphyrinogenic potential of new drugs. Although most such drugs are lipid-soluble, no common chemical or steric property has been identified, and the site of combination of such drugs and the nature of the biochemical lesion are unclear. No unifying hypothesis exists linking drug structure and biochemical lesion, and there is no way of predicting which new drugs are likely to be porphyrinogenic. Studies in experimental animals and in vitro cell systems have shown some consistency with the clinical situation, but clear correlation has so far eluded the scientists researching in this field.

FURTHER READING

Eales L (1979) Porphyria and life-threatening drugs. S Afr Med J 56:914
Disler P et al. (1982) Drugs in porphyrias. S Afr Med J 61:656
Moore MR (1980) Review of drugs in acute porphyria. Int J Biochem 12:1089

4 Drug Injuries

4.1 Drug Fever

Drug fever can be regarded as a febrile reaction resulting directly or indirectly from the administration of a therapeutic agent.

CAUSES

The most commonly reported causes are:
Blood products
Vaccines
Antibiotic and antituberculous agents
Sulphonamides
Antineoplastic agents
α-Methyldopa

The fever that may develop during the course of treatment of syphilis with penicillin, or with neuroleptic, anticholinergic and anaesthetic agents, is referred to below.

PATHOGENESIS

Three pathogenetic types of drug fever are recognised:

i) Fever resulting from drug hypersensitivity. This is the commonest type. Fever may occur alone, or in association with other allergic manifestations such as urticaria, serum sickness, hepatic dysfunction, haematological or bone marrow disturbance, and vasculitis.

ii) Fever resulting from the pharmacological action of the drug itself, e.g. the Herxheimer reaction, which is a consequence of the effect of penicillin on the spirochaetes in a patient with syphilis, or the fever associated with haemolysis in patients whose red blood cells are genetically deficient in glucose-6-phosphate dehydrogenase following administration of primaquine. Drugs such as phenothiazines may act on the central nervous system (usually in toxic doses) to cause fever by decreasing heat loss and increasing heat production.

iii) Fever resulting from the introduction of micro-organisms or pyrogens, or the development of a non-infected inflammatory response at the site of injection.

When drug fever in humans is due to an immunological mechanism, other features are often identifiable, viz:

i) Evidence of previous sensitisation with the drug, or closely related agent;
ii) An accelerated response upon readministration;
iii) The reaction is drug-specific;
iv) The clinical manifestations resemble those usually associated with immunological reactions; and
v) The reaction is not attributable to the pharmacological action of the drug.

The antigen may be the drug itself, a complex of drug and host protein, a degradation product, or a complex of host protein and degradation product. In the majority of drug allergies the precise immunological mechanism is undetermined. More than one immunological response may occur together, and different reactions may be noted simultaneously.

CLINICAL FEATURES

Two patterns of presentation are recognised: immediate onset, directly after administration of the offending agent, and delayed onset, 7–10 days or more after start of therapy. In the latter, fever may be the sole manifestation, part of a serum sickness-type reaction, or associated with cutaneous or systemic signs of an allergic response.

With discontinuation of the agent concerned the fever should settle promptly within 24 h, unless it is part of a systemic reaction, or is due to the effects of long-acting metabolites or impaired excretion of degradation products. In such cases fever can take 4–5 days to settle. Regardless of the nature of the onset, drug fever may pursue a sustained or a remittent course. Normally it persists as long as the drug is administered.

If a patient has been previously sensitised, or has experienced a prior febrile reaction, re-exposure to the drug may cause the temperature to rise abruptly, sometimes with a chill. (Drug fever, when it has an allergic basis, follows the same chronology as that of serum sickness or the other classical allergic reactions.)

PREDISPOSING FACTORS

Patients with an allergic diathesis are potentially at risk of developing an allergic form of drug fever, but there is no evidence that hay fever and bronchial asthma predispose to it. Genetic factors may be important and, as in the case of other antigens, the age of the patient, duration of exposure, dosage and route of administration and previous contact with closely related antigens may undoubtedly influence the frequency and nature of the reaction.

DIAGNOSIS

Drug fever should be regarded as a warning sign of an impending severe reaction, although in many instances it may remain the only manifestation of drug allergy. Fever is a common premonitory finding in serious adverse drug reactions such as anaphylaxis, agranulocytosis, aplastic anaemia, thrombocytopenic purpura, encephalopathy, and vasculitis.

The only direct evidence of a drug aetiology is the rapid development of fever following administration, prompt cessation on discontinuation of the drug and recrudescence upon subsequent readministration. Serological tests, skin tests and in vitro laboratory studies yield equivocal and inconsistent results.

Drug fever is suspected whenever a temperature which is unexpected and not attributable to the underlying disease process or to complications develops during a course of therapy.

MANAGEMENT

All medication should ideally be discontinued immediately the diagnosis is made. If the underlying disease is such that discontinuation of all drugs is unwise, drugs may be stopped one at a time, with a wait of 2–3 days in each instance to observe whether the fever abates. If simultaneous discontinuation of all drugs results in a good response, the responsible agents may be identified (if this is essential) by readministration of test doses of each, one at a time. However, such an approach can be dangerous, and should only be followed when the drugs concerned are required for a life-threatening condition, in the absence of suitable therapeutic alternatives.

If it is essential that therapy be continued with an agent responsible for a pyrexial reaction, this may be achieved by simultaneous administration of corticosteroids. These serve to suppress fever and other manifestations of drug allergy. Antihistamines may control manifestations such as mild urticaria, but they are ineffective in fever. Desensitisation with the offending drug yields inconsistent results, and success is usually transient. This approach has little to offer and it may be dangerous.

HERXHEIMER REACTION

The Herxheimer reaction classically occurs in patients with syphilis being treated with penicillin; it appears to be due to release of endotoxins from large numbers of killed organisms. The condition is not uncommon. Most prominent is fever, characteristically developing 6–8 h after initiation of therapy, and associated with myalgia and tachycardia. Symptoms should settle within 12–24 h, although patients with advanced cardiovascular or cerebral syphilis may deteriorate further, and fatal reactions have been recorded.

A similar reaction may occur with penicillin therapy of other infections, such as leptospirosis, yaws, rat-bite fever and anthrax.

MALIGNANT HYPERTHERMIA

This is a comparatively rare complication of potent inhalational anaesthetics such as halothane, and skeletal muscle relaxants. The clinical features are usually dramatic and severe: rapid onset of hyperpyrexia up to 42°C, rigors, tachycardia, cyanosis and muscle rigidity. Severe lactic acidosis, hyperkalaemia and acute renal failure often result, and the mortality of severe forms of the condition is of the order of 70%. The presentation may be mild, and a subclinical myopathy detected by raised creatine phosphokinase (CPK) levels in the serum may be the only finding.

An autosomal dominant genetic predisposition to this condition has been demonstrated. There may be a family history of the condition, and relatives at risk may be identified by raised CPK levels in the serum. The postulated genetic abnormality is abnormal muscle calcium storage, with massive calcium release following the pharmacological trigger.

NEUROLEPTIC
MALIGNANT SYNDROME

This is discussed in the section on neuroleptic agents (see p. 176).

FURTHER READING

Cluff LE, Johnson JE (1964) Drug fever. Prog Allergy 8:149
Lipsky BA, Hirschmann JV (1981) Drug fever. JAMA 245:851
Orme M (1977) Adverse reactions caused by drug metabolites. Adverse Drug Reaction Bull No 64:224

4.2 Anaphylaxis and Anaphylactoid Reactions

Acute anaphylaxis is an overwhelming allergic reaction to an antigen, usually mediated by IgE antibodies, and characterised by abrupt onset within seconds to hours after exposure. It mostly follows parenteral administration of antigenic drugs, but in extremely sensitive individuals it may be initiated by oral, topical or respiratory contact.

The terms "anaphylactoid" and "anaphylactic" are sometimes used interchangeably for such reactions; the clinical presentation of the two is indistinguishable. An anaphylactoid response can be regarded as the response developing on first exposure to an allergic agent, while anaphylaxis can be regarded as the subsequent event.

PATHOGENESIS

Penicillin is the major iatrogenic cause of systemic anaphylaxis. The estimated incidence in humans is about 1 per 4 000–10 000 injections, with fatality from 1 in every 100 000–500 000 doses. Other well-recognised drug causes of anaphylaxis are indicated in Table 4.1.

Table 4.1. Iatrogenic causes of anaphylaxis

Penicillin and congeners (including cephalosporins)
Vaccines[1]
Local anaesthetics[2]
Diagnostic agents for intravenous administration[3]
Ethylene oxide[4]
Aspirin, and other non-steroidal anti-inflammatory agents[5]
Aminoglycoside antibiotics

Notes:

1. These include diphtheria, pertussis, influenza, typhoid, mumps, measles, typhus, rabies and yellow fever vaccines. (Certain reactions involving viral vaccines appear to be due to sensitivity to egg proteins from the chick embryos used to propagate the virus.)

2. Cross-allergenicity exists between the various local anaesthetics. Anaesthetics of the amide type (bupivacaine, cinchocaine, lignocaine, mepivacaine, prilocaine) are safer than those of the ester type (amethocaine, benzocaine, cocaine, oxybuprocaine, procaine) with respect to the risk of allergic reactions.

3. These are usually low molecular weight compounds, such as organic iodides used in radio-opaque contrast media, non-iodine radiodiagnostic agents for intravenous administration, and sulphobromophthalein (BSP).

4. Residual traces of ethylene oxide used for sterilising plastic tubing or syringes for intravenous injections may cause severe systemic reactions.

5. Cross-sensitivity exists between related non-steroidal anti-inflammatory agents. Conversely, congeners of an anti-inflammatory agent responsible for anaphylaxis need not necessarily be anaphylactigenic themselves.

The precise role of histamine or other chemical mediators in human anaphylaxis is not clear. Slow-reacting substance A (SRS-A) may contribute to the bronchoconstriction. It is not known whether kinins or other pharmacologically active mediators take part in the reaction.

SYMPTOMATOLOGY

The acute response of the respiratory system characteristically develops within minutes of the antigenic challenge. A feeling of generalised warmth and tightness of the throat precedes wheezing and dyspnoea. Hypoxia, with cyanosis, may develop. Oedema of the hypopharynx, epiglottis, larynx and trachea may be severe enough to cause respiratory obstruction. Laryngeal oedema is suspected if there is hoarseness or stridor, or a sensation of a lump in the throat. Lower respiratory manifestations include wheezing and acute bronchospasm, with prolongation of expiration. Hyperinflation of the lungs is apparent in post-mortem studies of patients dying from anaphylaxis.

Several systems may be involved simultaneously, or the manifestations may be limited to a single organ. Generalised urticaria or angioedema are common. Localised urticarial lesions are frequently noted at the site of injection of the offending antigen, which may provide a clue to diagnosis. Nausea and vomiting, pruritus, palpitations, and a sensation of impending doom are early symptoms. Hypotension, arrhythmias and cardiac arrest may develop. Female patients may experience uterine cramping. Syncopy is relatively common and convulsions occasionally occur. Focal neurological manifestations are unusual.

The reaction time and syndromes of acute and subacute allergic drug manifestations are depicted in Fig. 4.1.

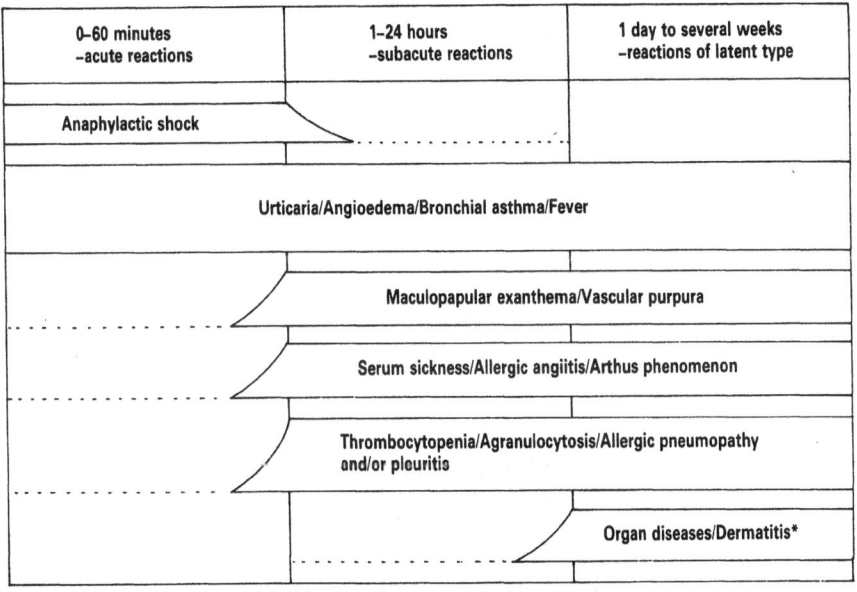

*from locally applied or ingested contact allergens

Fig. 4.1. Reaction time and anaphylactic and related syndromes [reproduced with permission from Hoigne et al. 1980].

PREDICTION AND
PREVENTION

Allergy to haptene drugs is idiosyncratic. For this reason, anaphylactic responses are not readily predictable, and it is often impossible to anticipate them. However, a profile of the patient at special risk can be defined, and the risks diminished, if not eliminated:

i) A patient with a history of drug hypersensitivity is in danger of developing an acute hypersensitivity response on subsequent re-exposure to the drug or a related antigen. (Drugs for which a known cross-sensitivity exists are indicated in Table 4.2.) Evidence of the existence of drug hypersensitivity is based on a relatively fixed induction period before the onset of symptoms in the first event (2–6 weeks), fever, skin rash, peripheral blood eosinophilia, and the demonstration (where appropriate) of non-caseating granulomas on liver biopsy. In practice, only a history of fever and skin rash will be available in most cases, and any account of such reaction indicates the necessity for great caution, and the patient should be regarded as potentially allergic to the drug or drugs concerned.

Table 4.2. Drugs with known cross-allergenicity

Penicillins / cephalosporins
Local anaesthetics of the ester-type (amethocaine, benzocaine, cocaine, oxybuprocaine, procaine)
Non-steroidal anti-inflammatory agents including aspirin and salicylates
Sulphonamides / sulphonylureas
Aminoglycoside antibiotics (streptomycin, kanamycin, gentamicin, tobramycin, amikacin, neomycin, framycetin)
Skeletal muscle relaxants (d-tubocurarine, alcuronium, pancuronium, suxamethonium)

ii) In asthmatic patients it appears that the type and intensity of reaction may be influenced adversely, but there is no evidence that non-asthmatic atopic persons are at greater risk than others. This opinion is not universally accepted.

iii) A history of food "sensitivity" raises a high index of suspicion, although a relationship with drug hypersensitivity is not established.

iv) There is no convincing evidence that a family history of drug allergy or atopic disorders, or factors such as age, sex, race, occupation or geographic location predispose a person to anaphylaxis.

v) No advantage exists in performing skin testing to predict drug hypersensitivity. In extremely sensitive individuals even percutaneous testing may result in severe symptoms, and possibly fatality. An allergic response may be due to minor determinants or degradation products of the drug, rather than the parent drug itself. The risks and problems of false-positive reactions are reduced if skin testing is performed with pure components (such as penicilloyl-polylysine in the case of penicillin), but this approach reduces the sensitivity of the test.

Anaphylactic deaths from penicillin occur less commonly from oral than parenteral administration. This is probably the case for other drugs as well. The reasons for the difference are likely to include slower absorption, differences in the antigenic nature of the formulations, destruction of antigen in the upper gastrointestinal tract, and failure of the gut to absorb macromolecular impurities.

In practice, the risks of anaphylaxis are reduced by taking a careful history of previous reactions with possible cross-reactants, the use of "medic-alert" tags to identify sensitive patients, strict avoidance of unnecessary or repeated therapy with highly immunogenic products, and the use of preparations, routes of therapy and dosage schedules with the least likelihood of causing reactions. In the patient for whom a potentially anaphylacti-genic drug may be life-saving and for whom no alternative is available, rapid intravenous desensitisation with progressively increasing doses may be required. This has to be carried out with corticosteroids and resuscitation facilities immediately available.

DIFFERENTIAL DIAGNOSIS This is considered in Table 4.3.

HOIGNE'S SYNDROME An acute, non-allergic, pseudo-anaphylactic reaction of varying severity is recognised in association with penicillin depot preparations (Hoigne's syndrome). The symptoms include confusion, acoustic and visual hallucinations, palpitations and cyanosis. Generalised seizures or twitches of the extremities are common. There is no cardiovascular collapse, distinguishing the reaction from anaphylaxis. The onset is sudden, occurring at the time of injection or a few seconds afterwards. As a

Table 4.3. Differential diagnosis of acute anaphylactic drug reactions

Condition	Comment
Acute vasovagal response to the trauma of injection of a drug or vaccine	Cutaneous and respiratory manifestations are absent; hypotension is moderate and there is a prompt response to recumbent position and reassurance
Acute pulmonary embolism. Acute myocardial infarction or cardiac arrhythmia	The differential diagnosis may be difficult in patients who are already critically ill, or receiving anaesthesia
Acute life-threatening reactions in patients with phaeochromocytoma, systemic mastocytosis or urticaria associated with C_1-esterase deficiency	The reaction may closely simulate anaphylaxis. The diagnosis is usually suggested by the history
Acute laryngeal obstruction due to infection, aspiration, foreign body or neurological disease	–
Acute embolic-toxic reaction to injected drugs (Hoigne's syndrome)	See text

rule the symptoms diminish and disappear within minutes to an hour. A minority of patients complain of milder symptoms for weeks or months. This reaction may be more common than is generally appreciated; with procaine penicillin the frequency may be 2–3 per 1000 injections.

The pathogenesis is not known. Affected patients do not have a history of allergy, and in a number penicillin has been administered subsequently without adverse effects. High systemic levels of procaine released from the depot preparation may cause neuropsychiatric effects. However, similar symptoms have been noted with procaine-free penicillin. At autopsy crystals of penicillin have been demonstrated in the lungs. An embolic-toxic response to accidental intravenous penetration or diffusion of procaine penicillin is the most likely explanation.

SERUM SICKNESS
REACTIONS

Serum sickness was originally described as a reaction to foreign serum, but today the syndrome is most commonly caused by drugs. Low molecular weight drugs are most commonly responsible (Table 4.4). Any macromolecules capable of causing anaphylaxis can also produce serum sickness. This suggests that the response in either case is due to direct protein reactivity of the host, or metabolic conversion of the offending agent to antigenic products. Serum sickness is an immune complex disease, with antigen excess in the

Table 4.4. Drugs associated with serum sickness-like reactions[a]

Penicillin, and cephalosporins[b]
Sulphonamides
Thiouracils
Hydantoins
Para-aminosalicylic acid
Penicillamine
Phenylbutazone
Cholecystographic dyes
Thiazide diuretics
Streptomycin

Notes:

[a]In approximate order of frequency.
[b]The cephalosporins are occasionally cross-allergenic with penicillins (approximately 20% overlap).

presence of antibody. The antibodies are mainly of the IgG class. Circulating complexes fix complement and deposit in small blood vessels and on the basement membrane of renal glomeruli. The role played by complement in the deposition of immune complexes is uncertain. The deposition of immune complexes appears to be related to changes in vascular permeability and homeostatic mechanisms influencing such permeability. Vasoactive mediators derived from basophils, mast cells and platelets play a role in the pathogenesis of serum sickness. The tissue damage is by a Type III hypersensitivity mechanism (see Fig. 4.2).

The target organs in serum sickness and the clinical patterns are indicated in Table 4.5. Characteristically the disease develops 8–10 days after antigen challenge, corresponding to maximum immune complex formation. An accelerated form may be seen hours after contact (differentiation from an acute anaphylactic response may not be possible in such cases). A delayed form may occur weeks after the initial antigenic challenge has ceased. Symptoms may be mild and last only a few hours, or severe and last for weeks; the usual course is several days to a week after the drug is withdrawn. This complication of drug therapy is probably more common than is widely appreciated.

CLASSIFICATION OF
ALLERGIC DRUG
REACTIONS

See Fig. 4.2. and the accompanying notes.

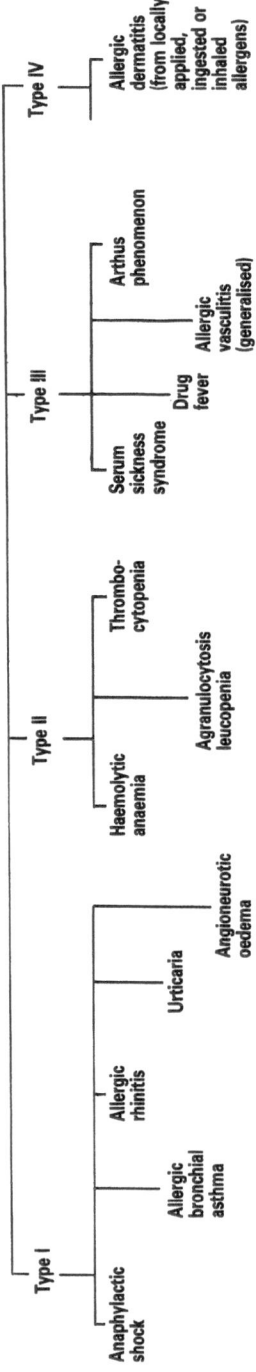

Fig. 4.2 Allergic drug reactions.

Notes to Fig. 4.2:

1. The classification is based upon that of Coombs RRA and Gell PGH (1968) Clinical aspects of immunology, 2nd ed. Blackwell, Oxford, p. 575.
2. In practice the proof that any one of these mechanisms is responsible for individual conditions may be impossible.
3. Mixed-type reactions frequently occur.
4. Examples of adverse reactions where classification of reaction type is not possible include macular and maculopapular exanthemas, exfoliative dermatitis, toxic epidermal necrolysis, vascular purpura, coagulopathy due to acquired inhibition of factor VIII, fixed drug eruptions, transient eosinophilic pulmonary infiltration, hepatitis, active chronic hepatitis, interstitial nephropathy, encephalitis, polyradiculitis (neuritis), LE-cell phenomenon, pancytopenia and "leukaemoid reaction".
5. Type I, II and III reactions are largely dependent upon the presence of circulating antibodies (and are in the broader sense compatible with reactions of the immediate type). Type IV reactions are based upon the presence of sensitised lymphocytes and are the actual "delayed type" hypersensitivity reactions.
6. The reaction time and type of immunological mechanism frequently do not coincide.

Table 4.5. Target organs and clinical patterns in serum sickness reactions

Organ	Clinical Pattern
Skin and mucous membranes[a]	Urticaria, maculopapular rash, oedema, vasculitis, angioneurotic oedema. Exfoliative dermatitis and Stevens-Johnson syndrome may occur. Erythema nodosum is uncommon. Polyarteritis nodosa is described
Lymph nodes and spleen[a]	Enlargement of lymph nodes. The spleen may be enlarged. (These findings are explained by a cellular proliferative response to antigenic stimulation)
Kidneys	Albuminuria and hyaline casts in the urine. Glomerulonephritis and/or interstitial nephritis may result
Joints	Painful, swollen joints; arthralgia
Myocardium	Myocarditis
Peripheral nerves[b]	Polyneuritis, mononeuritis or mononeuritis multiplex may develop, and rarely this dominates the clinical picture. The 5th cervical nerve root may be selectively involved, causing pain, paralysis and atrophy in that distribution

[a]Absence of skin rashes and lymphadenopathy militates strongly against the diagnosis.
[b]Mononeuritis and polyneuritis are thought to be due to perineural oedema, causing compression of nerve roots. Recovery is usually complete, but may take weeks or months.

FURTHER READING

Hoigne R et al. (1980) Penicillins, cephalosporins and tetracyclines. In: Dukes MNG (ed) Meyler's side effects of drugs, 9th edn. Excerpta Medica, Amsterdam, p 408
Kryst L, Wanyura H (1979) Hoigne's syndrome: its course and symptomatology. Maxillo-facial Surg 7:320
Miller KB et al. (1981) Rapid sensitisation for desferrioxamine anaphylactic reaction. Lancet I:1059

4.3 Drug-Induced Diseases of the Skin

Various important and common drug-induced disorders of the skin are indicated in Fig. 4.3. The list is not comprehensive and the inter-relationships which are indicated are tentative.

The skin is the largest organ of the body, and as such it is frequently involved in toxic and allergic drug reactions.

Notes to Fig. 4.3:

1. Acute and chronic urticarial syndromes are recognised. Women during their reproductive years are more likely to be affected than men, as a result of their greater cutaneous vascular lability. The essential lesion is leakage of protein from capillary vessels in a circumscribed area. The onset may be very rapid. It is regarded as a manifestation of immediate hypersensitivity mediated by histamine, serotonin, slow-reacting substance, etc., released as a result of direct or indirect drug injury.

2. Purpura is commonly associated with drug reactions. The primary damage may be to the capillary endothelium or the platelets, as a direct toxic effect, or in a type III or IV hypersensitivity response (see Fig. 4.2). Haemorrhage, lymphocyte infiltration and capillary necrosis may be associated with or progress to vasculitis.

3. Allergic vasculitis: see p. 171.

4. Photoallergic skin reactions are a form of contact dermatitis. Light transforms certain drugs into potent contact allergens. The wavelengths activating phototoxic responses are mainly in the ultraviolet region. Close similarity exists between photoallergic and ordinary contact allergic reactions, and they may be indistinguishable clinically and histopathologically. Erythema and oedema are the main clinical features.

5. Drugs particularly associated with erythema multiforme are penicillin, antipyretics, barbiturates, hydantoins and sulphonamides.

   The main pathological changes are lymphohistiocytic inflammatory infiltration around blood vessels, degenerative changes in endothelial cells of capillaries and papillary dermal oedema. An immune complex aetiology with hypocomplementaemic vasculitis is believed to be responsible. The syndrome may include systemic toxicity and high fever. Toxic epidermal necrolysis (Stevens-Johnson syndrome) is a severe mucocutaneous form of erythema multiforme.

6. See (5) above.

DIAGNOSIS AND NATURAL HISTORY

None of the skin reactions described in association with drugs can be regarded as pathognomonic of a drug aetiology.

Discontinuation of the responsible drug (dechallenge) can be expected to be followed by rapid disappearance of symptoms and signs. This may not be so when there is delayed excretion of the metabolites responsible for persistence of the reaction, when depot preparations are responsible, or when the patient is repeatedly exposed to the offending antigen (e.g. penicillin in milk).

Readministration of the drug or extracts of the antigen responsible (rechallenge) is normally but

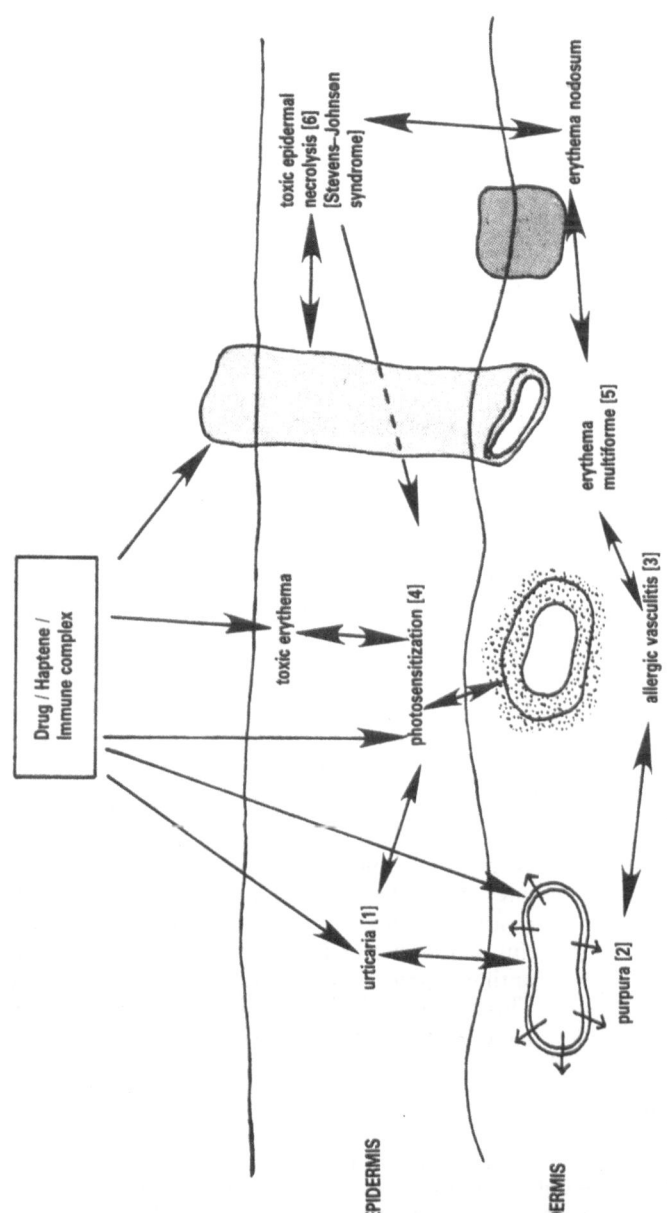

Fig. 4.3. Certain drug-induced skin diseases and their possible inter-relationships. (Numbers refer to the notes.)

not invariably associated with relapse. Rechallenge is rarely justified, as the effects can be catastrophic.

Skin testing to detect a drug thought to be responsible for a reaction is of little value when it has been given by another route. The allergen may be formed or released only after systemic administration. Fatal reactions have occurred to minute doses of antigen used in skin testing.

Various in vitro tests have been devised to confirm allergic reactions. These include the Prausnitz-Kustner (passive transfer) reaction, the direct and indirect basophil degranulation test, fluorometric assay of histamine release, lymphocyte transformation testing, enzyme-linked immunosorbent assay and others. Because of difficulties in performing the test, lack of reproducibility, and the possibility of the antigen being a derivative or metabolite formed in the body rather than the parent drug, these tests have not been found to be useful in practice.

The results of re-exposure to an antigen which has previously caused an adverse skin reaction are unpredictable, reflecting the lack of specificity and the versatility of the toxic skin response.

MANAGEMENT OF HYPERSENSITIVITY

Therapy with corticosteroids has not been effective in modifying the pathological response or the natural history of drug-induced skin disorders.

In a patient who has developed a drug-related skin reaction and who is in need of continued therapy, an agent chemically different from the offending one should be sought. If continued or repeated treatment with the responsible drug is essential, this should be carried out with corticosteroid and antihistamine cover, or desensitisation, or both. This would only be justified in situations where continued therapy is considered life-saving.

FURTHER READING

Calnan CD (1964) Urticarial reactions. Br Med J II:649
Criep LH (1967) Dermatologic allergy, diagnosis, management. Saunders, Philadelphia
Willis I, Kligman AM (1968) The mechanism of photoallergic contact dermatitis. J Invest Dermatol 51:378

4.4 Drug-Induced Vasculitis

Drugs are an important cause of allergic vasculitis (Table 4.6). Deposition of immune complex, which includes drug haptene, may be in arterioles, capillaries or post-capillary venules. There is evidence that the concentration of immune complex determines the site of vascular damage: high concentration may cause arterial involvement, while lower concentrations mainly affect capillaries and venules. Histamine plays a key role in vasculitic lesions in immune complex disease, directly acting on vessels and indirectly influencing localisation.

Table 4.6. Drugs causing hypersensitivity vasculitis

Allopurinol
Barbiturates
Diphenylhydantoin
Hydralazine
Iodine-containing dyes for radiodiagnosis
Oral contraceptives
Penicillamine
Penicillin
Phenylbutazone
Propylthiouracil
Salicylates
Sulphonamides

CLINICAL FEATURES

The clinical features and natural history of vasculitis are determined by the localisation and extent of involvement. When lesions are confined to venules symptoms result from local haemorrhage, exudation and micro-infarcts. More widespread disease is likely to include fever, erythema and maculopapular rashes, pneumonitis, albuminuria, haematuria, renal failure, neuropathy, and leucocytosis with eosinophilia. A particular target organ may be affected. Patients who die show evidence of focal or diffuse glomerulonephritis. Necrotising vasculitis may result in haemorrhage and ischaemia of multiple organs.

ALLOPURINOL
HYPERSENSITIVITY

Several aspects of the natural history of allopurinol hypersensitivity may have a bearing on other drug-related vasculitides:

i) The illness begins 4–6 weeks after commencement of therapy, suggesting that a period of sensitisation is required.

ii) Active disease appears to be temporally

related to the presence of circulating antigen.

iii) In severe cases there may be prolonged illness, lasting weeks or months after the drug has been discontinued. (A metabolite of allopurinol might provide a persistent antigenic stimulus. Alternatively, an immunological response directed against allopurinol or its metabolites could conceivably cross-react with normal purines, ribonucleotides or nucleic acids, resulting in an illness prolonged beyond the persistence of the original antigen.)

iv) Results of therapy with corticosteroids have been inconclusive.

v) Reactions have been worse and more common in patients with high plasma levels of the parent drug or metabolites. Reduction of renal function, in which the clearance of allopurinol and its metabolite, oxypurinol, is diminished, and concomitant therapy with thiazide diuretics, which compete with oxypurinol for renal tubular secretion and elimination, appear to increase the likelihood of this association.

vi) A generalised maculopapular eruption associated with pruritus, and sometimes exfoliation or bullus formation, is invariable in severely affected individuals.

vii) The cutaneous effects of severe vasculitis are frequently associated with hepatomegaly and abnormal liver function. Deterioration of renal function with oliguria and haematuria, and gastrointestinal bleeding are common features of generalised allopurinol vasculitis.

FURTHER READING

Al-Kawas FH et al. (1981) Allopurinol hepatotoxicity. Ann Intern Med 95:588
Greaves MW (1980) Pharmacological factors in initiation of cutaneous vasculitis. In: Wolff K, Winkelmann RK (eds) Vasculitis. Lloyd-Luke, London, p 49
McCombs RP (1965) Systemic allergic vasculitis. JAMA 194:1059

4.5 Drug-Induced Vomiting

Various drugs and toxins that influence the vomiting mechanism are indicated in Fig. 4.4. In general, the mechanism whereby most drugs cause vomiting is not well understood. The chemoreceptor trigger zone (CTZ), which is located in the area postrema in the floor of the fourth ventricle, is accessible from blood and cerebrospinal fluid and appears to be activated by chemical stimuli only. An array of different chemoreceptors in the CTZ mediate the effect of blood-borne drugs and toxins.

The proposed sites of action of the antiemetic agents are indicated in Fig. 4.4. Antiemetics acting on the emetic centre (atropine, some antihistamines) will affect vomiting from any cause, but drugs acting on the CTZ (phenothiazines, metoclopramide) only influence vomiting mediated via the chemoreceptors (e.g. morphine, digoxin).

Antiemetic drug activity on the emetic centre is probably due to an anticholinergic action and that on the CTZ is antidopaminergic. The antiemetic action of many antihistamines may be due to their anticholinergic actions.

METOCLOPRAMIDE

Metoclopramide is structurally related to procainamide. It acts on the CTZ at least partly through blockade of dopaminergic receptors. It also has a peripheral action increasing gastric peristalsis and emptying and relaxing the pyloric antrum and duodenal cap. The closing pressure of the lower oesophageal sphincter is raised. The actions of metoclopramide on the gastrointestinal tract are antagonised by atropine and other anticholinergics. Gastric secretion is not affected. Adverse reactions include extrapyramidal dystonia, such as occurs with phenothiazines. Metoclopramide stimulates prolactin release and may cause gynaecomastia and abnormal lactation.

CANNABINOIDS

Patients with refractory nausea and vomiting from cancer chemotherapy have been treated with Δ^9-tetrahydrocannabinol (THC). In several studies patients have shown a complete or partial response, often associated with temporary mood changes such as laughing, heightened awareness, elation, mild time distortion and pleasant hallucinations. Δ^9-Tetrahydrocannabinol or related chemical analogues may prove to have antiemetic activity in patients receiving chemotherapy, particularly in those who have failed to respond to

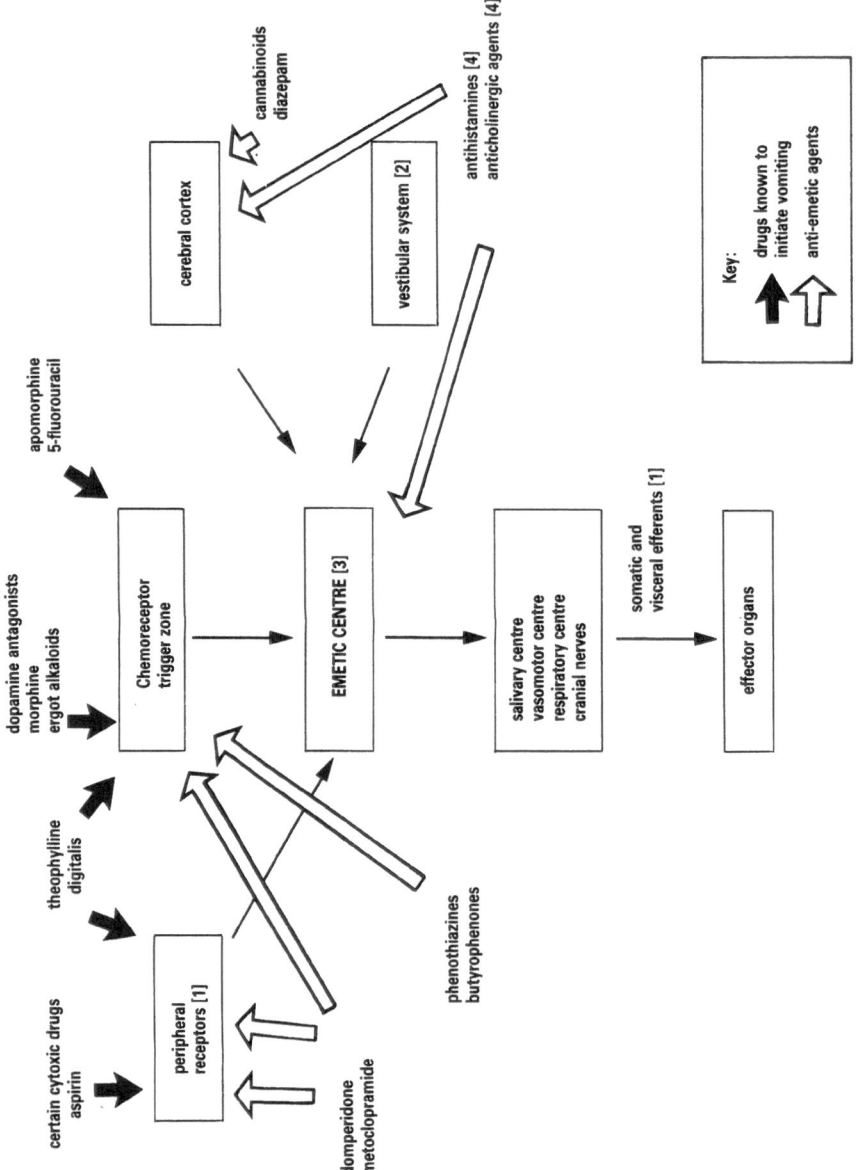

Fig. 4.4. Reflex pathways for vomiting and proposed sites of action of emetic and antiemetic agents.
Notes: 1. Refers to stomach, upper small intestine, peritoneum, genitourinary tract and spinal column. Gastric dopamine or opiate receptors may play an important role in mediating either the afferent or efferent limbs of the emetic pathway. 2. The vestibular centre is believed not to be important in pharmacologically mediated vomiting. 3. As far as is known no drug has a direct emetic action on the vomiting centre. 4. Proposed, but not substantiated.

standard therapy. This remains to be confirmed in controlled studies. The antiemetic effect of THC may depend upon the chemotherapeutic agents used (cisplatin-induced vomiting seems to be refractory to THC). The mechanism by which THC acts as an antiemetic is not known.

The use of the H_2-receptor blocking agents, non-steroidal anti-inflammatory agents, and opiate agonists and antagonists as antiemetic agents has not been properly evaluated.

FURTHER READING

Sallan SE et al. (1980) Antiemetics (THC) in cancer chemotherapy. N Engl J Med 302:135
Siegel LJ, Longo DL (1981) Control of chemotherapy-induced emesis. Ann Intern Med 95:352

4.6 Central Anticholinergic Syndromes

Anticholinergic drugs which act on the central nervous system (for example phenothiazines, butyrophenones, antihistamines and tricyclic antidepressants) may, under certain circumstances, cause central anticholinergic toxicity. Figure 4.5 depicts the pathogenesis and spectrum of central anticholinergic syndromes. Psychotic patients who receive potent neuroleptics, the geriatric population and alcoholics are a special risk category. Underlying organic brain disease may also be a predisposing factor in the pathogenesis of central anticholinergic syndromes, although this association has never been substantiated. These complications are more likely in patients taking two or more such agents simultaneously.

TOXIC CONFUSIONAL STATE	Confusion, agitation, restlessness and other features of an acute toxic confusional state may develop with centrally acting anticholinergic agents, not necessarily in conjunction with prominent peripheral anticholinergic manifestations. Psychosis, confusion, hallucinations, severe agitation, motor incoordination, dysarthria, ataxia and rigidity are results of large doses. Children and the elderly are at special risk. Potentially dangerous tachyarrhythmias may develop.
	Eye signs are unreliable as an indication of anticholinergic toxicity. Pupillary dilatation in a confused psychotic patient may be caused by excessive sympathetic discharge in response to

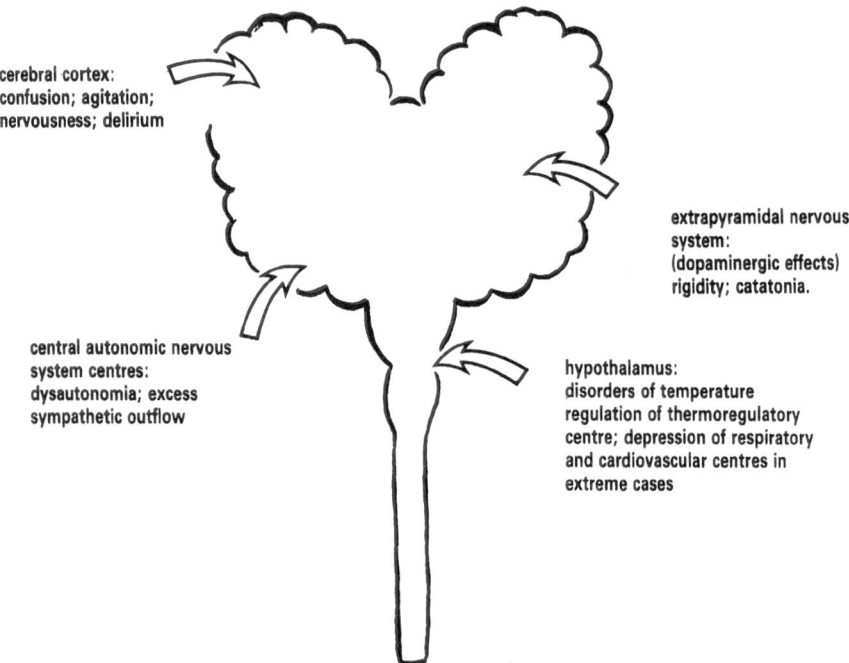

cerebral cortex:
confusion; agitation;
nervousness; delirium

extrapyramidal nervous
system:
(dopaminergic effects)
rigidity; catatonia.

central autonomic nervous
system centres:
dysautonomia; excess
sympathetic outflow

hypothalamus:
disorders of temperature
regulation of thermoregulatory
centre; depression of respiratory
and cardiovascular centres in
extreme cases

Fig. 4.5. Pathogenesis and spectrum of central anticholinergic syndromes

agitation, and in elderly subjects pupillary responses to drugs can be sluggish.

DISORDERS OF TEMPERATURE CONTROL

Large doses of centrally acting anticholinergic agents may render a patient poikilothermic as a result of a combined effect on (i) thermoregulatory control in the hypothalamus, (ii) inhibition of sweating due to a peripheral antimuscarinic effect, and (iii) cutaneous vasodilatation that may be due to α-adrenergic receptor blockade. Hypothermia in cold weather and heat stroke in subjects who are exposed to a high ambient temperature (climatic, underground activity, sauna baths, etc.) or who participate in sports in which excessive endogenous heat may be generated, such as long-distance running, are well documented.

NEUROLEPTIC MALIGNANT SYNDROME

The most severe presentation of this drug-related disturbance is the neuroleptic malignant syndrome (NMS). This is a rare and sometimes fatal consequence of high doses of dopamine-depleting and anticholinergic drugs. It is mainly associated with parenteral use in psychotic patients. The pathogenesis is not known; a combination of reduced central nervous system dopamine activity and peripheral inhibition of sweating with impaired cutaneous heat loss has been suggested. (Thermoregulation in experimental animals is believed to reside in dopaminergic nerve terminals of the hypothalamus.)

The clinical manifestations of the NMS are hyperthermia, peripheral anticholinergic symptoms, muscular rigidity, and various degrees of impairment of consciousness. The biochemical basis of the latter is not known. Severe extrapyramidal rigidity is always present, probably due to diminished function of dopaminergic neurones. Involuntary movements, pallor, sweating, salivation, tachypnoea, tachycardia and instability of the blood pressure are characteristic. Serum creatinine phosphokinase (CPK) is elevated, possibly caused by disruption of the contraction and relaxation mechanisms of skeletal muscles.

Not infrequently the NMS culminates in coma, severe dehydration and acute renal failure, and the estimated mortality is 25%.

Drug-related central anticholinergic syndromes are easily misdiagnosed, and their differentiation from myasthenia gravis and "lethal catatonia" may be difficult. The latter is an acute catatonic state with delirium, associated with muscle rigidity and hyperpyrexia. The clinical picture may be indistinguishable from the NMS, although descriptions of the syndrome antedated neuroleptic drug therapy.

PHYSOSTIGMINE

Physostigmine counteracts the central and peripheral anticholinergic effects of the phenothiazines, butyrophenones, antihistamines, and tricyclic antidepressants. Of the various anticholinesterases available for clinical use, physostigmine penetrates best to the central nervous system. Most authorities agree that physostigmine should be given to patients with life-threatening signs of acute anticholinergic overdosage, such as coma with respiratory depression, uncontrollable epileptic seizures or severe hypertension.

The efficacy of physostigmine is limited by its rapid metabolism (hydrolytic cleavage by cholinesterases), and there is a risk of severe cholinergic effects developing with excessive dosage. Bronchospasm, hypersalivation, increased respiratory secretions, bradycardia, severe hypotension and generalised convulsions may complicate the cholinergic hyperstimulation of intravenous administration. On the other hand, the drug's acute preganglionic stimulation of the adrenal glands may cause an acute sympathetic effect as a result of release of adrenaline and noradrenaline.

For these reasons, when active pharmacological intervention is deemed urgent, intramuscular rather than intravenous physostigmine is sometimes preferred. When symptoms recur repeated doses may be necessary.

There is little evidence that physostigmine is of value in cardiac dysrhythmias or conduction disturbances of acute anticholinergic poisoning, and it is not beneficial in the neuroleptic malignant syndrome.

FURTHER READING

Hall RC et al. (1981) Anticholinergic psychosis. Psychosomatics 22:581
Mann SC, Boger WP (1978) Psychotropic drugs. Am J Psychiatry 135:1097
Tune LE et al. (1981) Delirium associated with anticholinergic drugs. Lancet II:651

4.7 Drug-Induced Ototoxicity

The drugs most commonly responsible for ototoxicity are aminoglycoside antibiotics, salicylates and other non-steroidal anti-inflammatory agents, loop diuretics (frusemide and ethacrynic acid), certain cancer chemotherapeutic agents and antimalarials (Table 4.7).

The main toxic effect may be to the hearing mechanism or to the vestibular system, or both. Early damage is usually reversible, provided it is detected early and the offending agent is discontinued in time. Irreversible impairment of function may result from prolonged use.

The risk of ototoxicity is heightened when there is decreased renal function or pre-existing neurosensory hearing loss. The geriatric age group, being most likely to suffer from both of these, is especially vulnerable.

Table 4.7. Ototoxic drugs[a]

Antibiotics	Other drugs
Aminoglycosides	Chemotherapeutic agents:
Vancomycin	cisplatin
	nitrogen mustard
Diuretics	Salicylates
Frusemide	Non-steroidal anti-inflammatory agents
Ethacrynic acid	
	Antimalarials
	Quinine
	Chloroquine

[a]Combinations of these drugs are likely to increase the danger of ototoxicity.

DIAGNOSIS

Symptoms include tinnitus, hearing loss and vertigo, which may be associated with nystagmus.

To rely on tinnitus as a sign of ototoxicity can be misleading, as virtually all drugs have been associated with the complaint. Furthermore, advanced otic damage may occur without tinnitus being experienced.

The highest frequencies of hearing are lost first; subsequently lower frequencies are progressively involved, and finally all may be destroyed. In patients considered to be at particular risk pre-treatment audiograms and cold caloric vestibular testing should be performed. Unfortunately, audiometry often does not detect early hearing loss, and the severity of illness of patients receiving aminoglycoside antibiotics may preclude evaluation.

Daily questioning of the patient receiving potentially ototoxic drugs with regard to the symptoms of tinnitus, loss or alteration of hearing, and vertigo is essential. Development of these symptoms is an indication for audiovestibular testing and review of the treatment regimen.

AMINOGLYCOSIDES

Aminoglycoside antibiotics have been shown to concentrate in the perilymph of the inner ear, often in concentrations several times that found in the serum, and to persist many hours longer, particularly in patients with reduced renal function. Damage results from destruction of the receptor hair cells in the organ of Corti.

SALICYLATES   In high doses salicylates cause tinnitus and bilateral reversible neurosensory hearing loss. Therapeutic blood levels may impair hearing. The frequency characteristics of this hearing loss may take many forms, and the effects are normally reversible.

The effect of salicylates on the inner ear is not understood. The lack of evidence of structural abnormalities (even at the electron microscopical level) and the reversibility of the effect suggest an enzymatic mechanism.

NON-STEROIDAL ANTI-   These drugs have also been implicated in
INFLAMMATORY AGENTS   ototoxicity.

ANTIMALARIALS   Quinine and chloroquine have been associated with hearing loss.

LOOP DIURETICS   Frusemide and ethacrynic acid may cause auditory loss, proportional to dosage and more pronounced in patients with diminished renal function. The onset of symptoms is often sudden and the hearing disorder is usually transient, although permanent audiovestibular damage has been reported.

FURTHER READING

Nathan MD (1981) Drug-induced hearing loss in the elderly. Geriatrics 36:95

5 Diagnosing Adverse Drug Reactions

The documentation of adverse reactions to drugs (ADRs) should ideally include quantitation and qualification of the likelihood of association, of morbidity and severity, and of the contribution of underlying and precipitating causes. Improving the quality of such information is important for several reasons. In the first place, better medical care would be assured. Potentially avoidable drug-related problems would be more likely to be prevented, and the identification of new and unusual toxic drug effects would be facilitated. This is particularly true for those adverse drug effects which are difficult to distinguish from common, spontaneously occurring diseases. Finally, and increasingly, there are medicolegal necessities for developing this field of medicine.

CLASSIFICATION

An adverse drug reaction is an undesirable clinical manifestation consequent upon, and caused by, the administration of a particular drug.

A useful classification of ADRs has been set out by Rawlins and Thompson (see Further Reading). The merit of this approach is that it has implications for the quality of care. ADRs can be classified as two types:

Type A: Undesirable effects that are known to be associated with the drug concerned, and that occur routinely, or as a result of excessive dosage, or when there is increased sensitivity. Examples are codeine-related constipation, insulin hypoglycaemia, and nausea induced by morphine. Such reactions can be anticipated, and in some cases prevented. Reactions of this kind are comparatively common.

Type B: Idiosyncratic reactions, which occur less frequently, and which cannot normally

serious implications. Penicillin anaphylaxis, or agranulocytosis due to chloramphenicol or phenylbutazone are examples of idiosyncratic reactions. Vigilance
is essential to reduce the risks of these
reactions.

For most adverse reactions to drugs there is an
individual variation in response. In predictable
reactions this is accounted for mainly by pharmacokinetic factors, rather than by differences in
target organ sensitivity. Undefined genetic,
biochemical and immunological determinants
influence the incidence and manifestations of
idiosyncratic reactions. In all ADRs the relationship of the event with the drug dose is of
importance.

The common adverse reactions and the special
risk factors in their development are indicated in
Table 5.1.

The drugs most frequently involved in ADRs (in
approximate order of frequency) are indicated in
Table 5.2.

Table 5.1. Common ADRs in practice and special risk factors in their development

Common ADRs	Special risk factors
Cardiac arrhythmias	Old age
Allergic reactions	Impaired renal function
Haemorrhage	Previous history of ADR
Congestive cardiac failure	Malignant disease (cytotoxic drug therapy)
Bronchospasm	
Hypoglycaemia	

Table 5.2. Drugs most frequently involved in ADRs (in approximate order of frequency)

Digitalis
Antibiotics
Potassium supplements
Hypoglycaemic agents
Oral contraceptives
Anticoagulants
Diuretics
Antihypertensive agents
Analgesics
Corticosteroids
Phenolphthalein

PROBABILITY OF
ASSOCIATION

The criteria for causation of disease by an external agent (as laid down by the United States Surgeon General's Advisory Committee on Smoking and Health) can logically be applied to adverse drug reactions:

i) The association should be consistent, which implies that findings should be replicated when the association is studied in different localities and by different methods.

ii) The association should be a strong one. This refers to both the magnitude of the association and the existence of a dose-response relationship.

iii) The association should be "distinctive". In a distinctive association the relationship between the suspected agent and the effect should be specific for those two entities. The likelihood of a particular disorder being associated with a given aetiological agent is less if that disorder also frequently occurs in association with other conditions.

iv) There should be a temporal relationship between exposure to the alleged cause and development of the effect.

v) The association should be coherent, that is, it should be plausible according to "known facts in the natural history and biology of the disease".

The algorithm set out in Fig. 5.1 helps to define the degree of probability of association of a suspected ADR and to reduce confounding effects.

For several reasons defining such association for drug-related events may be problematic. The clinical situation may be so complex that drug effects may pass unnoticed. The most seriously ill patients are the most susceptible to severe adverse drug effects. Furthermore, drugs may have a "nocebo" effect quite unrelated to their pharmacological action or toxicity, which may make the diagnosis of a toxicological effect more difficult. Nocebo effects include headache, nausea, dizziness, rash and fever. There may be an absence of clear temporal relationship between drug and clinical event such as in the case of oestrogen-related carcinoma of the vagina developing years later in the

	-2	-1	0	+1	+2
1. Previous experience With the drug[a]		☐	☐	☐	☐
2. Alternative aetiological candidates[b]	☐	☐	☐	☐	
3. Timing of events[c]		☐	☐	☐	
4. Drug levels and evidence of overdose			☐	☐	
5. Dechallenge		☐	☐	☐	
6. Rechallenge		☐	☐	☐	

Scoring: Range -7 to +7

+7 or +6 —probability of ADR is definite
+5 or +4 —an ADR is probable
+3, +2, +1 or 0 —ADR is possible
less than 0 —an ADR is unlikely

Key: +1 = evidence clearly favours an ADR   +2 = absence of any alternative aetiological candidates
0 = evidence is insufficient, equivocal or contradictory   -2 = timing of events is inconsistent with an ADR
-1 = evidence is clearly against a diagnosis of ADR

[a] Refers to whether or not the observed clinical manifestation has ever been reported with the suspected drug, and whether or not it is recognised as occurring as a consequence of the administration of the drug.

[b] This weighs other possible causes of the clinical manifestation (e.g. underlying disease, new illness, non-drug therapeutic effect, diagnostic tests or procedures.)

[c] Probability is rated according to the time of appearance of the clinical manifestation relative to the administration of the suspected drug.

Notes:

1. When a patient is receiving more than one drug suspected of causing a clinical manifestation, each possible paired combination of drug and clinical manifestation should be submitted to the algorithm and scored separately. (i.e. when several drugs are being taken the algorithms can be used to determine which one is the most likely cause of the observed clinical manifestation).

2. With minor modifications this algorithm can be adapted to assess ADRs to drug withdrawal and adverse drug–drug interactions.

3. When ADRs are considered as such only when they are regarded as definite or probable the true incidence is underestimated; if "possible" ADRs are included the incidence tends to be overestimated.

Fig. 5.1. Probability of association of an adverse clinical event with a drug (based on Naranjo et al. 1981).

daughters of mothers who received the hormone during pregnancy. When drugs cause subclinical toxicity, such as renal or hepatic biochemical effects only, the difficulties of establishing the association are considerable. All these reasons make it important that proper controls are established in evaluating ADRs. This implies measuring the suspected effect both in association with the drug and without it. Diagnostic difficulties arise when one of several drugs may be responsible for a drug-related event, when a reaction is odd or bizarre and not commonly recognised as being associated with a drug, or when the drug effect simulates a commonly occurring disease.

SEVERITY

Adverse drug reactions often tend to be reported with little attention given to their importance or the degree of morbidity. Tallarida et al. (1979) have given a lead in assessing and describing the severity of ADRs (Fig. 5.2).

1   Mild disease/effect; symptoms not progressive (e.g. mild headache, hay fever).

2   More severe than (1) (e.g. severe headache.)

3   Chronic effect; may interfere with normal activity, or incapacitating for intermittent periods of time (e.g. bronchial asthma, epilepsy)

4   Chronic disease, incapacitating but not considered life-threatening or life-shortening

5   Shortens life expectancy, but not considered life-threatening (e.g. hypertension)

6   Considered life-threatening (in 1–2 years), but not a medical emergency.

7   A disease or condition which is considered a medical emergency or which is likely to terminate life within 1 year or less, (e.g. severe cardiac arrhythmia, acute anaphylaxis)

Fig. 5.2. A scale for assessing the severity of adverse drug reactions (based on Tallarida et al. 1979)

BERKSON'S BIAS

An important source of bias in considering adverse reactions to drugs is the extrapolation of hospital-derived data to the non-hospital patient population. Berkson recognised that in comparing disease incidence in a hospital population with the incidence of the same disease in the population served by the hospital, bias is likely to be introduced as a result of co-morbidity presentations, which are more likely to be found in hospitalised patients. It follows that comparable details of incidence and severity do not necessarily apply to situations other than where they are studied.

It is important that patients at high risk of drug toxicity should be identified as far as this can be achieved.

FURTHER READING

Jones JK (1979) Assessment of adverse drug reactions in the hospital setting. Hospital Formulary 14:769

Kramer MS (1981) Difficulties in assessing the adverse effects of drugs. Br J Clin Pharmacol 11:1055

Naranjo CA et al. (1981) A method for estimating the probability of adverse drug reactions. Clin Pharmacol Ther 30:239

Rawlins MD, Thompson JW (1977) Pathogenesis of adverse drug reactions. In: Davies DM (ed) Textbook of adverse drug reactions. Oxford University Press, Oxford

Roberts RS et al. (1978) An empirical demonstration of Berkson's bias. J Chron Dis 31:119

Surgeon General's Advisory Committee on Smoking and Health (1964) Criteria for causation of disease. Public Health Service Publication No 1103, US Department of Health Education and Welfare, Washington DC

Tallarida RJ et al. (1979) A scale for assessing the severity of diseases and adverse drug reactions. Clin Pharmacol Ther 25:381

Subject Index

P. I. Folb

The Safety of Medicines

Evaluation and Prediction

Foreword by J. R. Trounce
1980. 4 figures, 7 tables. XII, 103 pages
ISBN 3-540-10143-8

Contents: Animal Testing and Early Studies in Humans. – Prediction of Teratogenic Potential or a New Medicine. – Prediction of Dependence-Producing Potential of A New Drug. – Prediction of Carcinogenic Potential of a New Medicine. – The Prediction of Adverse Drug Interactions. – Monitoring Drug Safety in Clinical Practice. – Subject Index.

Physicians and pharmacists have become increasingly aware that, among the unprecedentedly large number of new drugs introduced in the last thirty years are many which may at times contribute to the morbidity of their patients. This book defines guidelines for judging independently the safety of medicines based on preclinical animal research and clinical data from early human studies. Principles for weighing the practical problems of drug dependence, teratogenesis, drug-induced allergic reactions, haematological and biochemical aberrations, adverse drug-drug interactions, and drug-induced carcinogenesis are considered in detail. The strength and limitation of prospective and retrospective clinical studies and drug monitoring and reporting systems in the diagnosis of adverse drug reactions are examined. A case is made for reducing, wherever possible, unnecessarily tedious, expensive and wasteful animal experimentation, with recommendations made for simpler, more economic means of evaluating medicines.

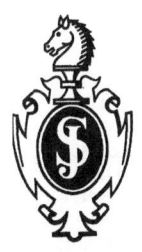

Springer-Verlag
Berlin
Heidelberg
New York
Tokyo

H. Capell, T. J. Daymond, W. C. Dick

Rheumatic Disease

1983. Approx. 5 figures, approx. 47 tables. Approx. 210 pages
(Treatment in Clinical Medicine)
ISBN 3-540-12622-8

Contents: Introduction. – General Principles and Approach to the
Patient in the Context of Osteoarthritis. – Pain in the Neck, Low
Back Pain and Degenerative Disc Disease. – Local Syndromes. –
Metabolic Bone Disease. – Crystal Arthropathies. – General Medi-
cal and Metabolic Diseases. – Rheumatoid Disease and Manage-
ment of Extra-articular Features. – Juvenile Chronic Arthritis. – The
Seronegative Spondarthritides. – Infective Arthritis and Polymyalgia
Rheumatica/Giant Cell Arthritis. – Connective Tissue Disorders. –
The General Principles of Management of Chronic Arthritis. – Phar-
macology of the Drugs Used in the Treatment of Chronic Arthritis.
– Gold. – Penicillamine. – Antimaterials and Other Possible-Line
Drugs. – Corticosteroids. – Surgery. – Subject Index.

Rheumatic Disease deals with the drug treatment of these disorders
within the context of their overall management. There are two
broad sections. The first discusses various diagnoses briefly and
gives details of the approach to management. The second section
gives more comprehensive information about individual drugs and
emphasises those which are either peculiar to rheumatology or are
especially relevant to patients with rheumatological diseases. In
addition to background information, a practical guide to the use and
potential toxicity of these preparations is provided.

Gastrointestinal Disease

Editor: **C. J. C. Roberts**

1983. Approx. 3 figures, approx. 21 tables. Approx. 240 pages
(Treatment in Clinical Medicine)
ISBN 3-540-12531-0

Contents: Oesophageal Disease. Peptic Ulcer Disease. The Malab-
sorption Syndrome. Infective Diarrhoea. Inflammatory Bowel
Disease. The Irritable Bowel Syndrome and Diverticular Disease.
Disease of the Biliary System. Hepatic Disease. Pancreatic Disease.
Tropical Diseases Affecting the Gastrointestinal Tract and Liver. –
Clinical Pharmacological Considerations. Drug Toxicity in the
Gastrointestinal Tract and Liver. Nutritional Support in Gastrointe-
stinal Disease. Drugs for Gastrointestinal Disease. – Subject Index.

Gastrointestinal Disease, the first volume in the series, comprises 14
chapters and is divided into two sections. The first section is devoted
to the treatment of common disorders in the gastrointestinal tract,
liver and pancreas and includes a chapter on tropical diseases. The
second covers the clinical pharmacology of drug treatment in
gastroenterology and includes practical advice on systems for nutritional support.

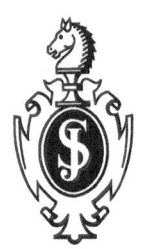

Springer-Verlag
Berlin
Heidelberg
New York
Tokyo